The Mediterranean Soups and Stews Recipe Book

Simple and Tasty Recipes to Enjoy Soups and Stews and Boost Your Diet

Fern Bullock

Table of Contents

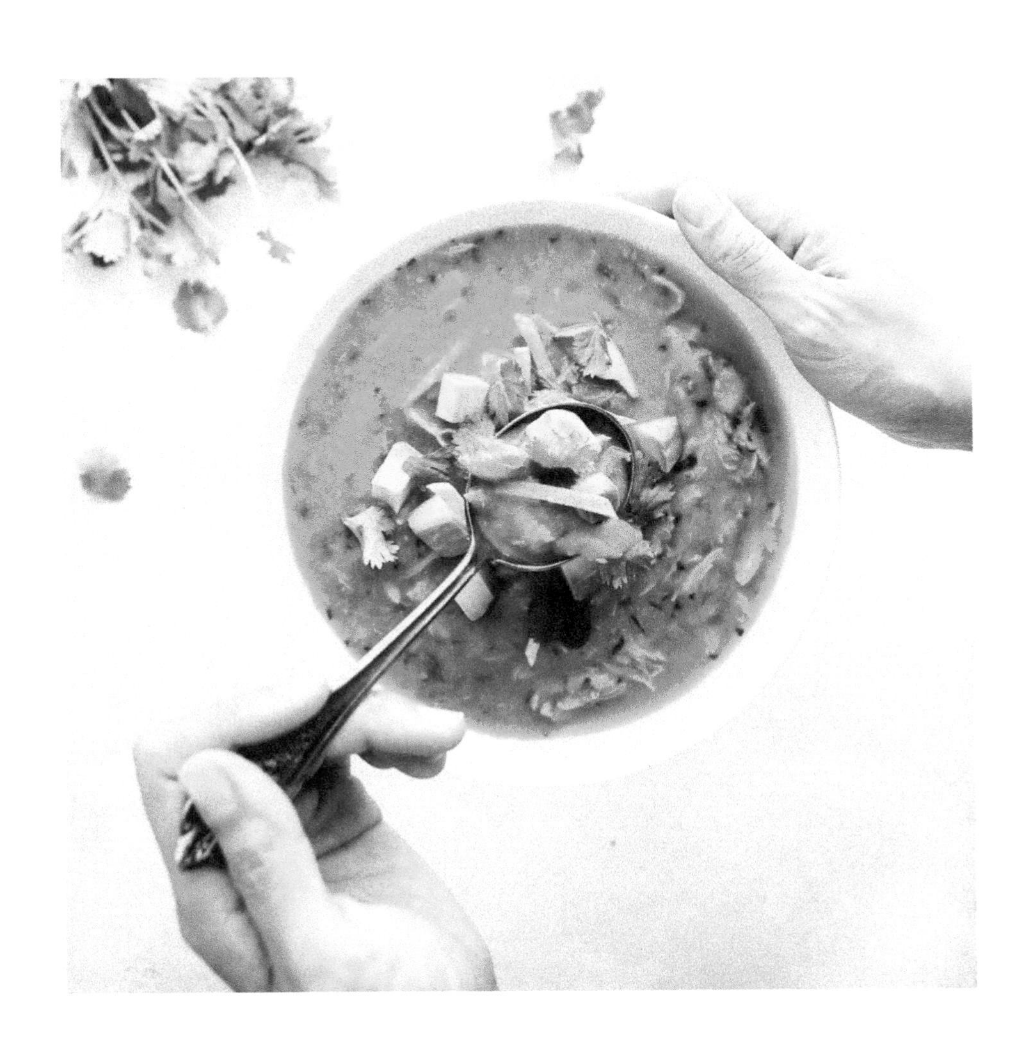

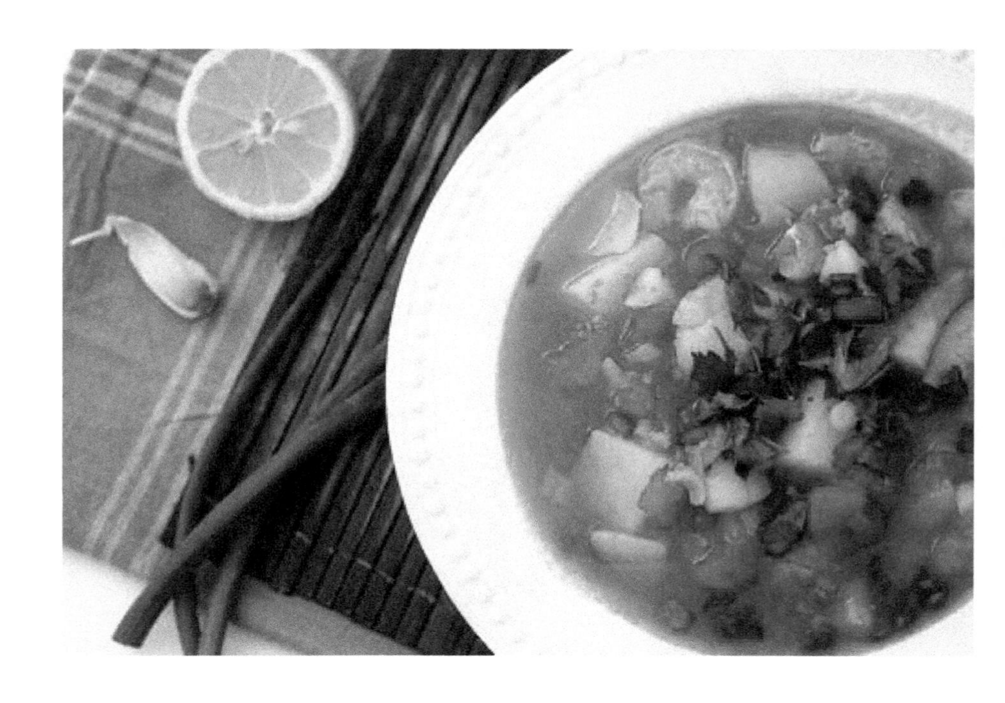

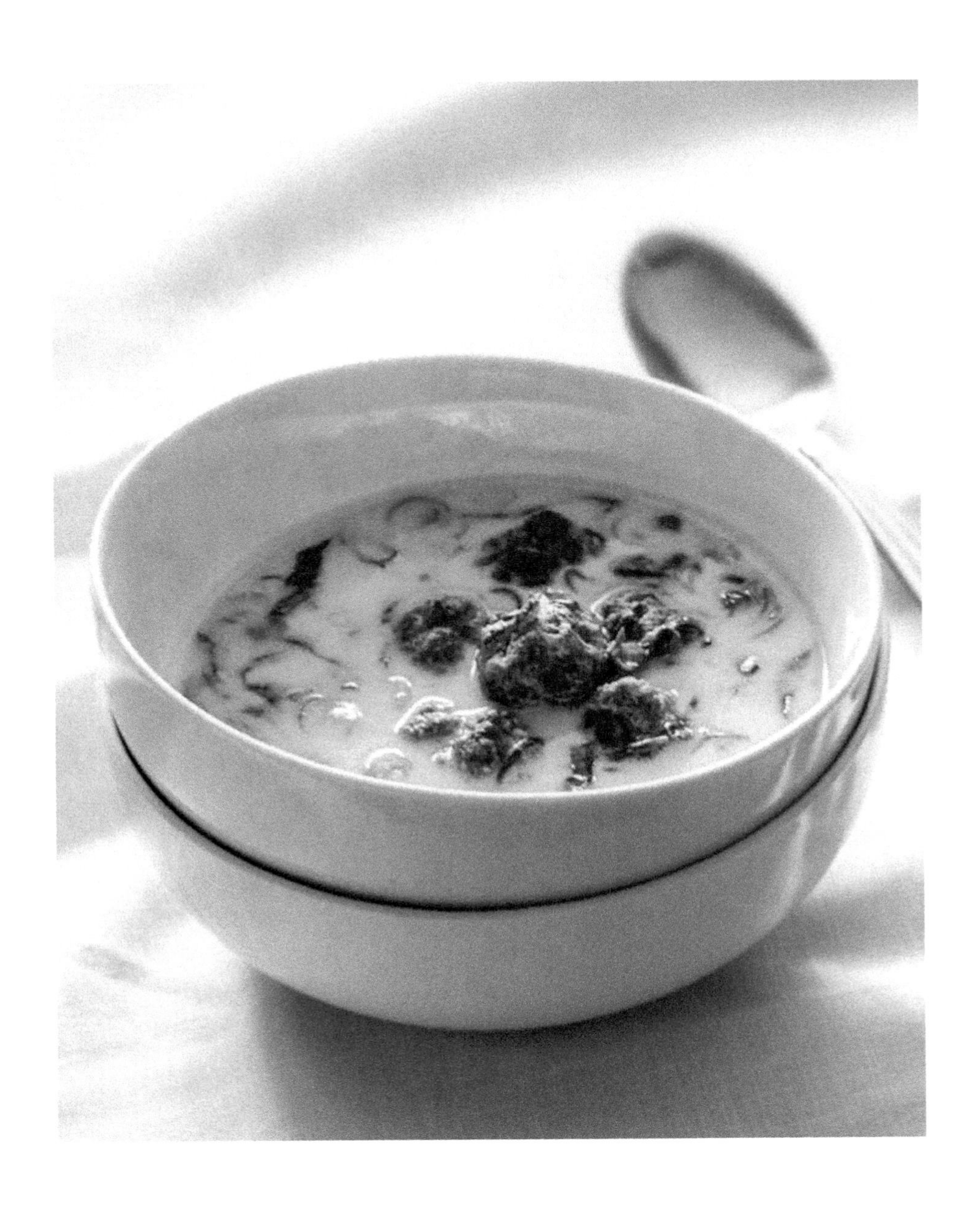

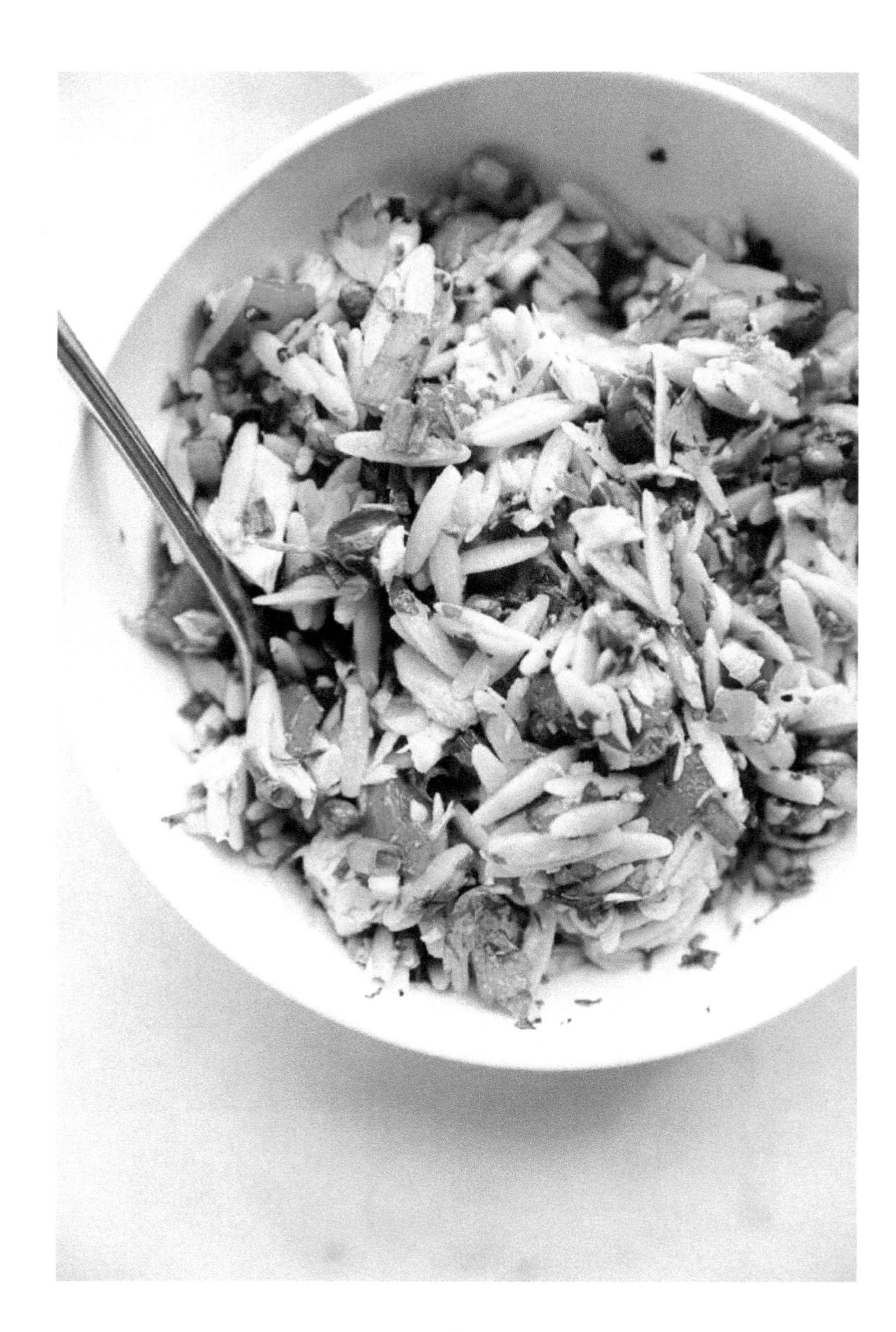

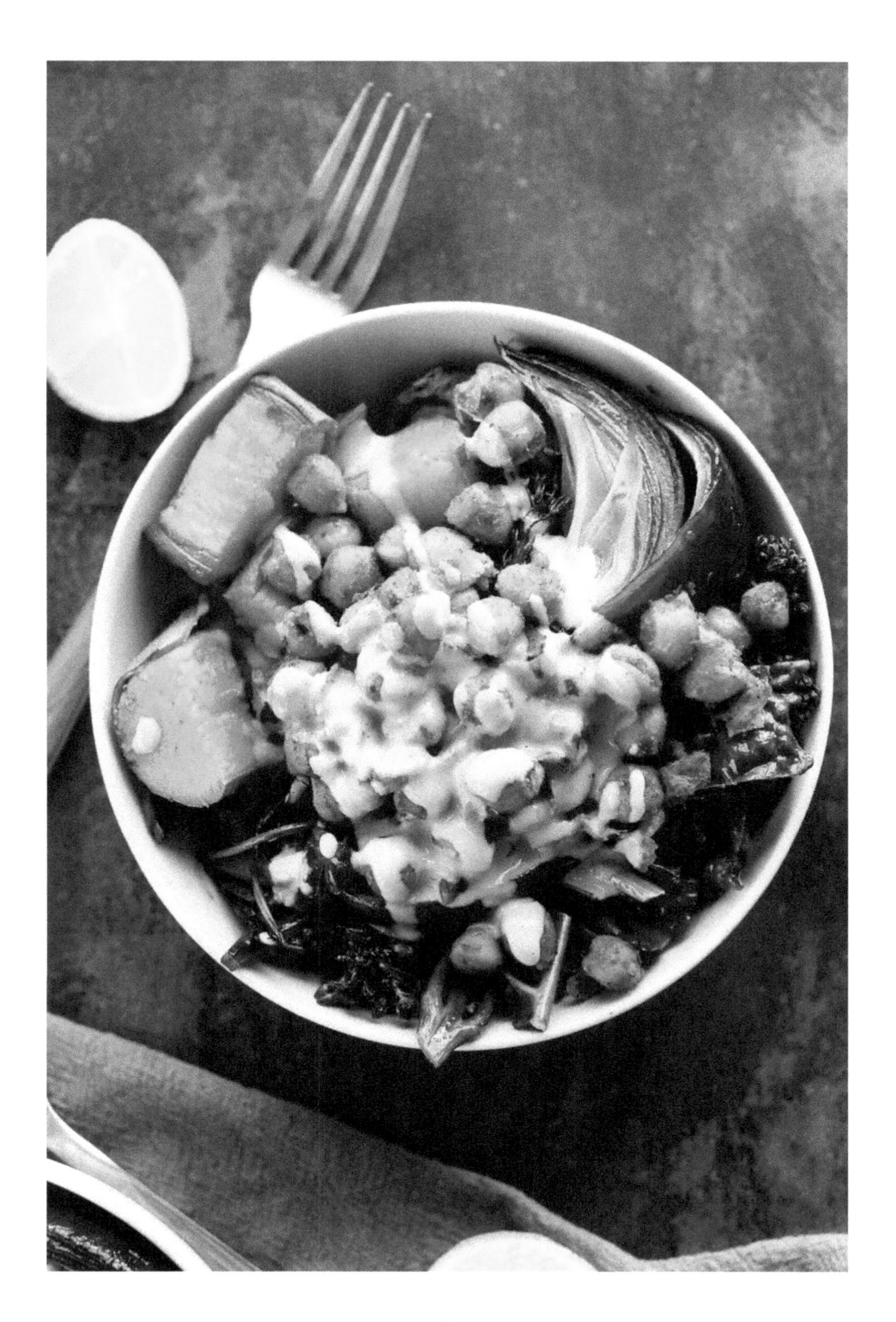

Shrimp and Orange Mix

Prep time: 5 minutes I **Cooking time:** 0 minutes I **Servings:** 4

Ingredients:

- 1 orange, peeled and cut into segments
- 1 pound shrimp, cooked, peeled and deveined
- 2 cups baby arugula
- 1 avocado, pitted, peeled and cubed
- 2 tablespoons olive oil
- 2 tablespoons balsamic vinegar
- Juice of½ orange
- Salt and black pepper

Directions:

1. In a salad bowl, mix combine the shrimp with the oranges and the other ingredients, toss and serve for lunch.

Nutrition facts per serving: calories 300, fat 5.2, fiber 2, carbs 11.4, protein 6.7

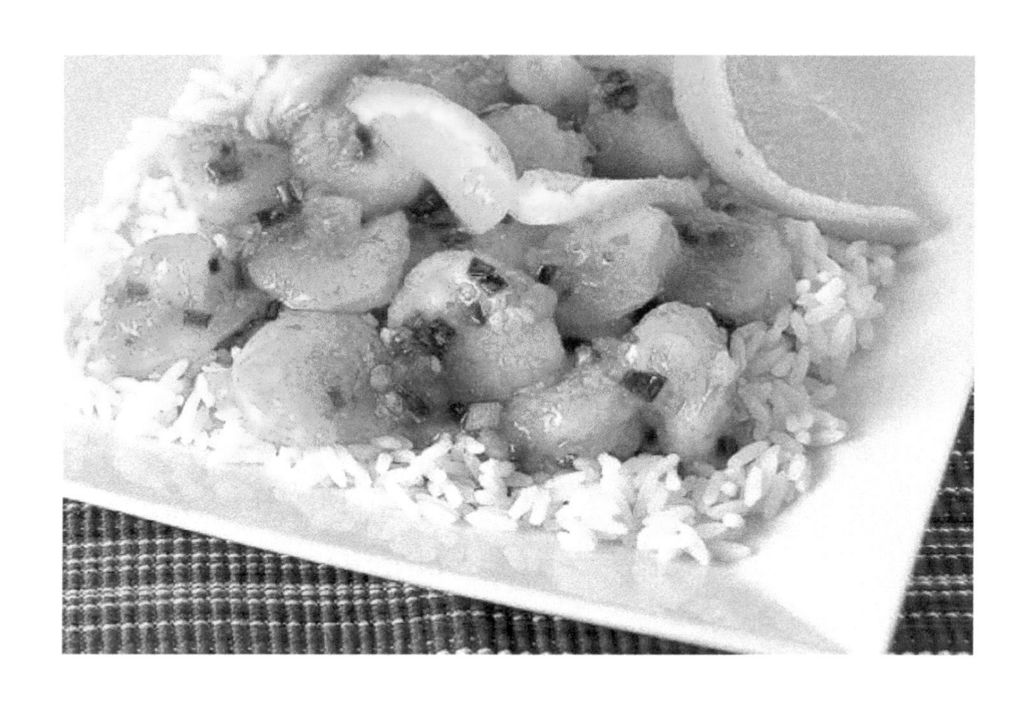

Broccoli Soup

Prep time: 10 minutes I **Cooking time:** 40 minutes I **Servings:** 4

Ingredients:

- 2 pounds broccoli florets
- 1 yellow onion, chopped
- 1 tablespoon olive oil
- Black pepper to the taste
- 2 garlic cloves, minced
- 3 cups beef stock
- 1 cup coconut milk
- 2 tablespoons cilantro, chopped

Directions:

1. Heat up a pot with the oil over medium heat, add the onion and the garlic, stir and sauté for 5 minutes.
2. Add the broccoli and the other ingredients except the coconut milk, bring to a simmer and cook over medium heat for 35 minutes more.
3. Blend the soup using an immersion blender, add the coconut milk, pulse again, divide into bowls and serve.

Nutrition facts per serving: calories 330, fat 11.2, fiber 9.1, carbs 16.4, protein 9.7

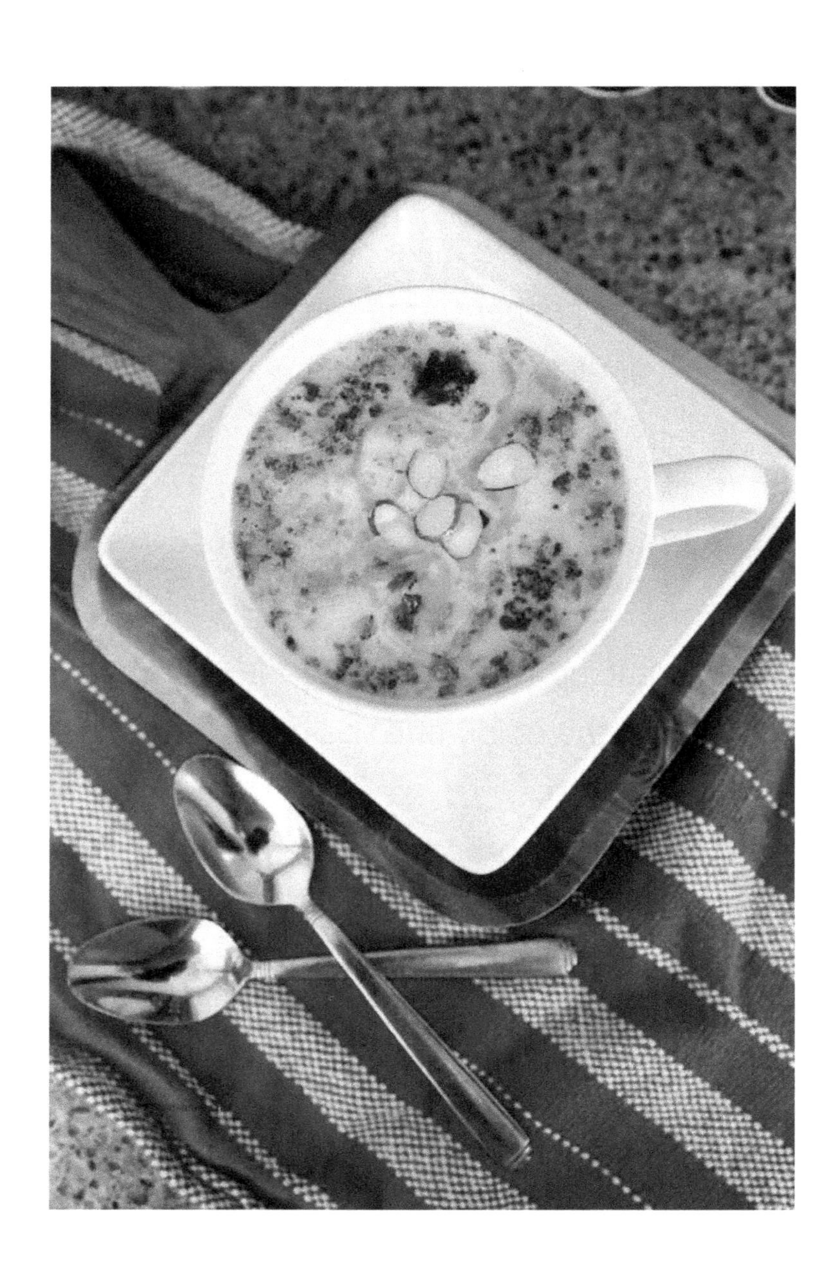

Cabbage, Leek and Tomato Soup

Prep time: 10 minutes I **Cooking time:** 40 minutes I **Servings:** 4

Ingredients:

- 1 big green cabbage head, roughly shredded
- 1 yellow onion, chopped
- 1 tablespoon olive oil
- Black pepper to the taste
- 1 leek, chopped
- 2 cups tomatoes, chopped
- 4 cups chicken stock
- 1 tablespoon cilantro, chopped

Directions:

1. Heat up a pot with the oil over medium heat, add the onion and the leek, stir and cook for 5 minutes.
2. Add the cabbage and the rest of the ingredients except the cilantro, bring to a simmer and cook over medium heat for 35 minutes.
3. Ladle the soup into bowls, sprinkle the cilantro on top and serve.

Nutrition facts per serving: calories 340, fat 11.7, fiber 6, carbs 25.8, protein 11.8

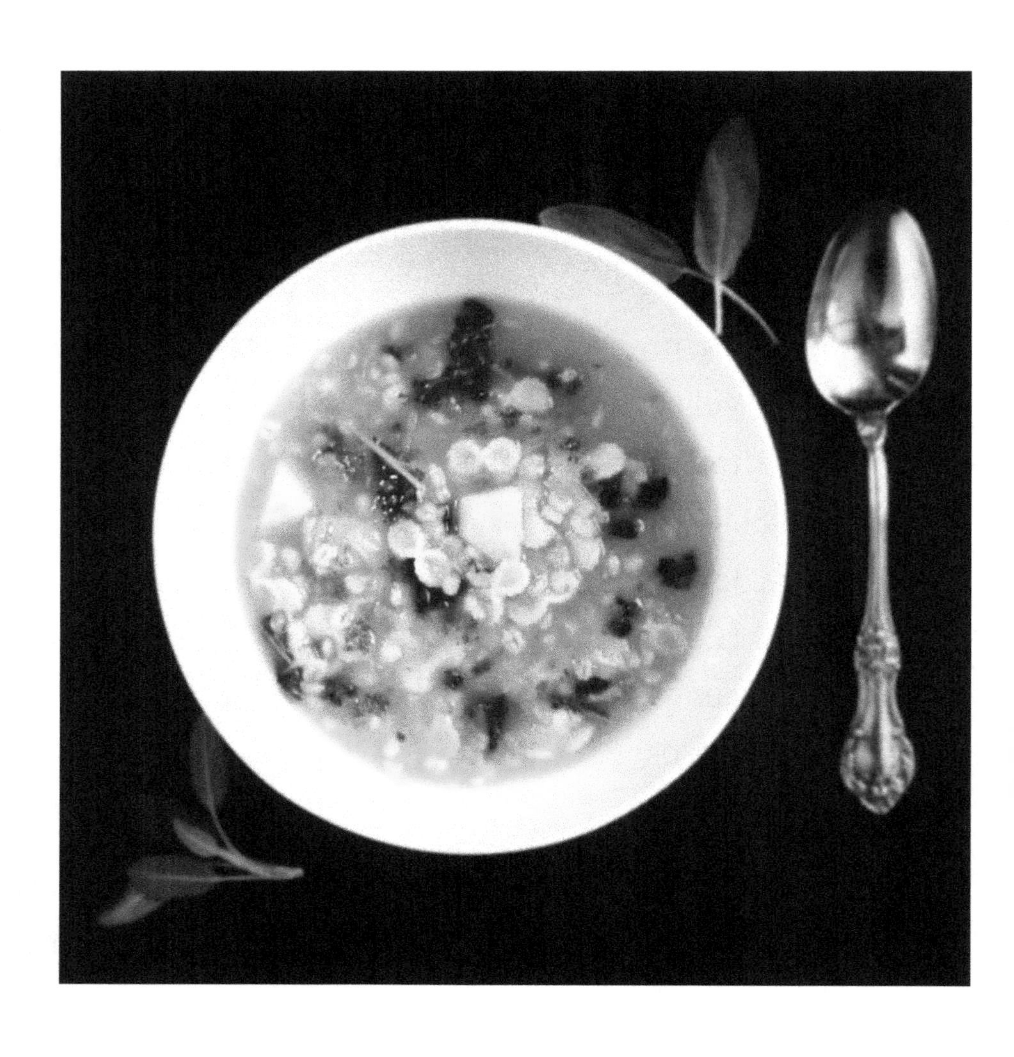

Cauliflower Soup

Prep time: 10 minutes I **Cooking time:** 40 minutes I **Servings:** 4

Ingredients:

- 2 pounds cauliflower florets
- 1 red onion, chopped
- 1 tablespoon olive oil
- 1 cup tomato puree
- Black pepper to the taste
- 1 cup celery, chopped
- 6 cups chicken stock
- 1 tablespoon dill, chopped

Directions:

1. Heat up a pot with the oil over medium-high heat, add the onion and the celery, stir and sauté for 5 minutes.
2. Add the cauliflower and the rest of the ingredients, bring to a simmer and cook over medium heat for 35 minutes more.
3. Divide the soup into bowls and serve.

Nutrition facts per serving: calories 135, fat 4, fiber 8, carbs 21.4, protein 7.7

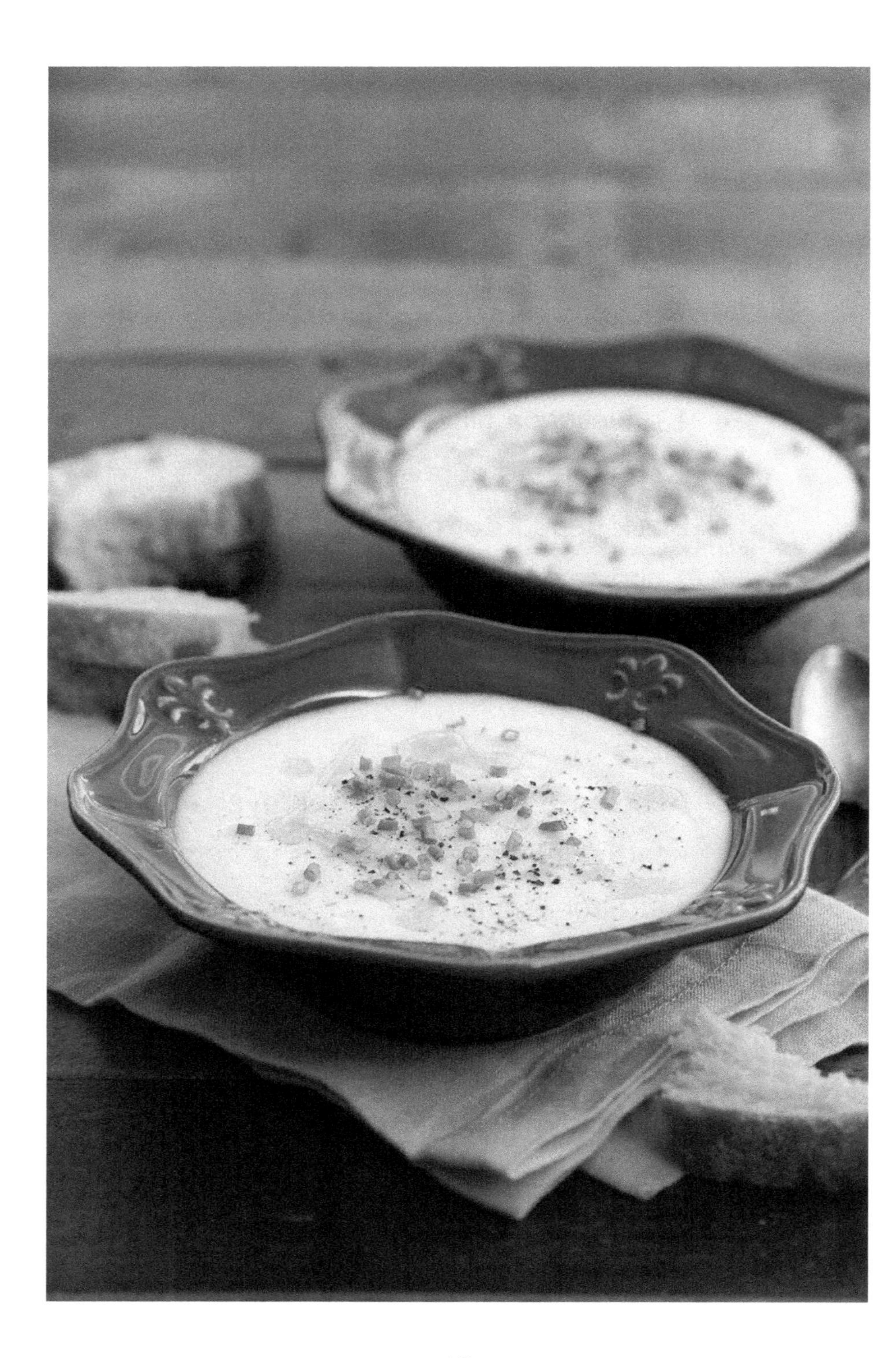

Parsley Pork and Leeks Soup

Prep time: 10 minutes I **Cooking time:** 40 minutes I **Servings:** 4

Ingredients:

- 1 pound pork stew meat, cubed
- Black pepper to the taste
- 5 leeks, chopped
- 1 yellow onion, chopped
- 2 tablespoons olive oil
- 1 tablespoon parsley, chopped
- 6 cups beef stock

Directions:

1. Heat up a pot with the oil over medium-high heat, add the onion and the leeks, stir and sauté for 5 minutes.
2. Add the meat, stir and brown for 5 minutes more.
3. Add the rest of the ingredients, bring to a simmer and cook over medium heat for 30 minutes.
4. Ladle the soup into bowls and serve.

Nutrition facts per serving: calories 395, fat 18.3, fiber 2.6, carbs 18.4, protein 38.2

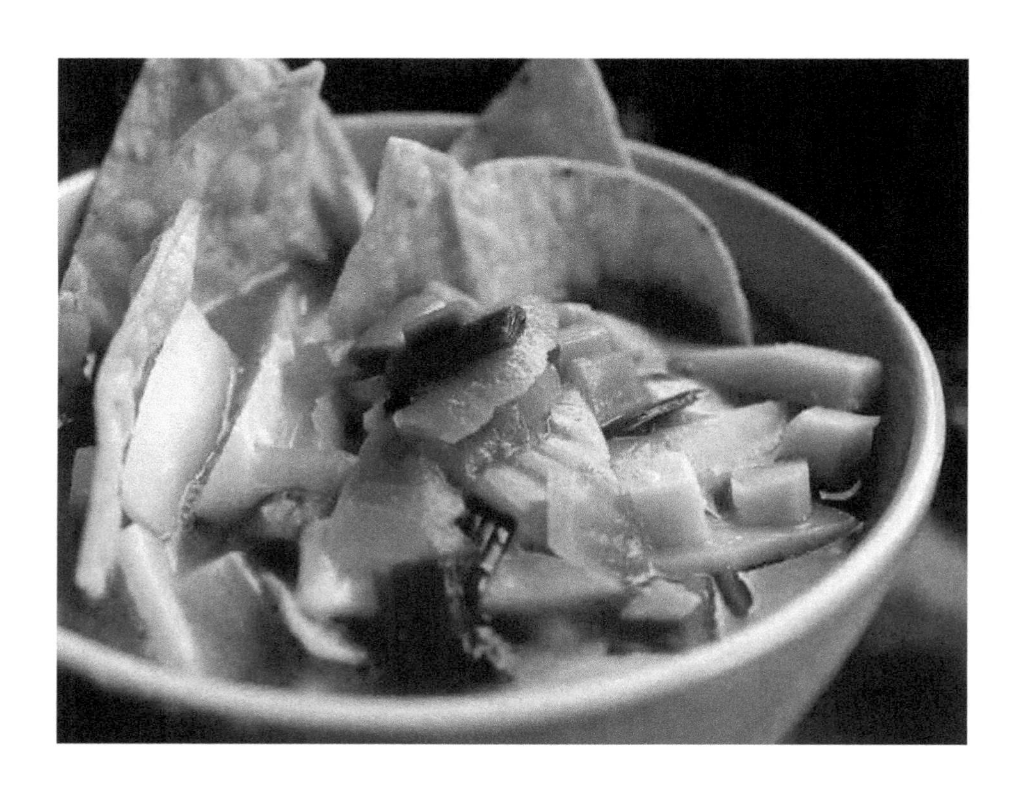

Shrimp and Broccoli Salad

Prep time: 5 minutes I **Cooking time:** 20 minutes I **Servings:** 4

Ingredients:

- 1/3 cup veggie stock
- 2 tablespoons olive oil
- 2 cups broccoli florets
- 1 pound shrimp, peeled and deveined
- Black pepper to the taste
- 1 yellow onion, chopped
- 4 cherry tomatoes, halved
- 2 garlic cloves, minced
- Juice of ½ lemon
- ½ cup kalamata olives, pitted and cut into halves
- 1 tablespoon mint, chopped

Directions:

1. Heat up a pan with the oil over medium-high heat, add the onion and the garlic, stir and sauté for 3 minutes.
2. Add the shrimp, toss and cook for 2 minutes more.
3. Add the broccoli and the other ingredients, toss, cook everything for 10 minutes, divide into bowls and serve for lunch.

Nutrition facts per serving: calories 270, fat 11.3, fiber 4.1, carbs 14.3, protein 28.9

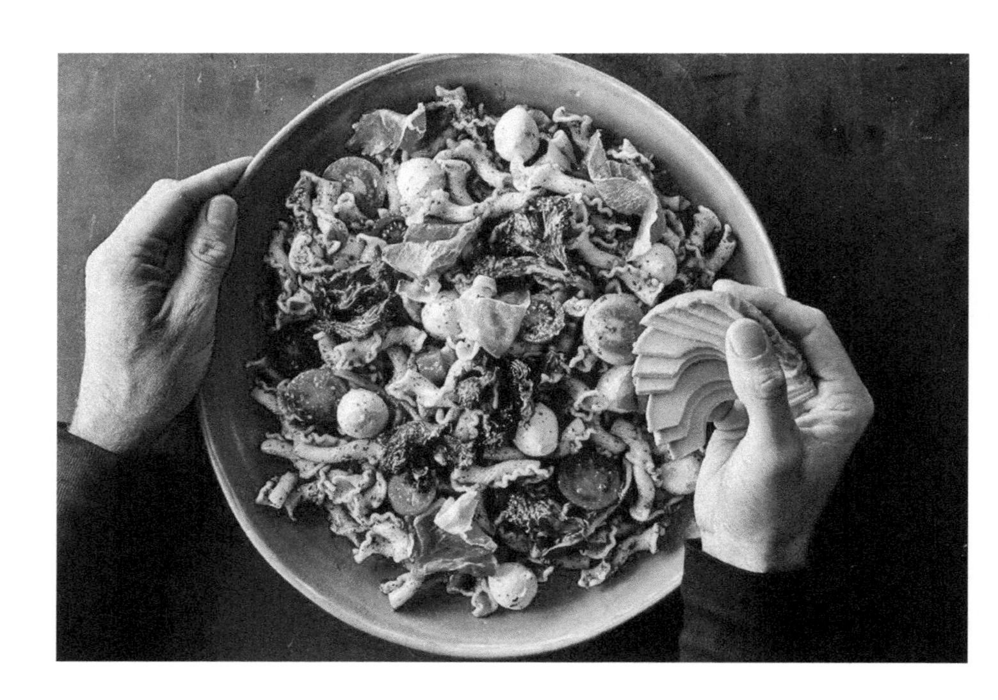

Chili Shrimp Soup

Prep time: 10 minutes I **Cooking time:** 20 minutes I **Servings:** 4

Ingredients:

- 1 quart chicken stock
- ½ pound shrimp, peeled and deveined
- ½ pound cod fillets, boneless, skinless and cubed
- 2 tablespoons olive oil
- 2 teaspoons chili powder
- 1 teaspoon sweet paprika
- 2 shallots, chopped
- A pinch of black pepper
- 1 tablespoon dill, chopped

Directions:

1. Heat up a pot with the oil over medium heat, add the shallots, stir and sauté for 5 minutes.
2. Add the shrimp and the cod, and cook for 5 minutes more.
3. Add the rest of the ingredients, bring to a simmer and cook over medium heat for 10 minutes.
4. Divide the soup into bowls and serve.

Nutrition facts per serving: calories 189, fat 8.8, fiber 0.8, carbs 3.2, protein 24.6

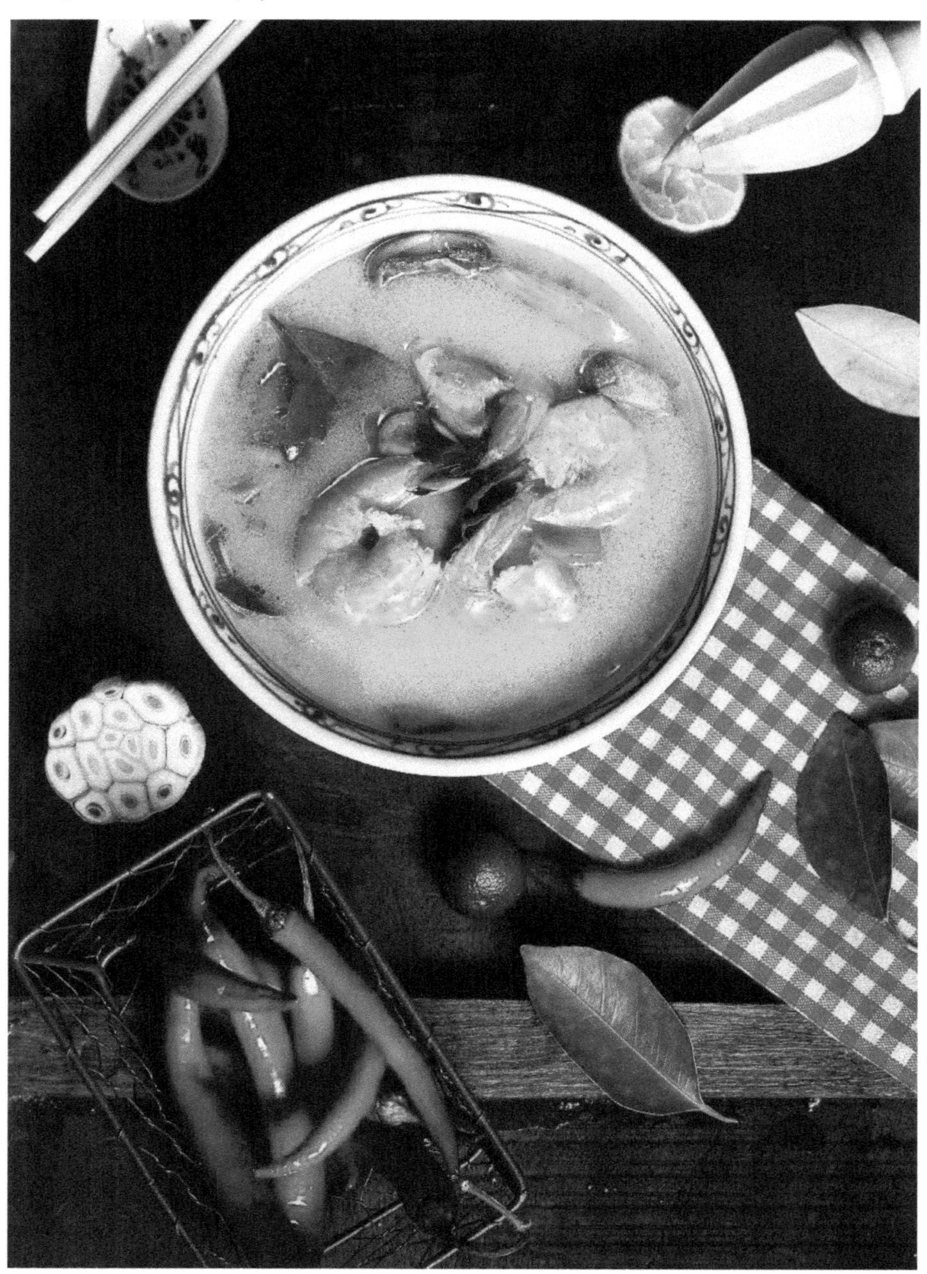

Shrimp, Onions and Tomato Mix

Prep time: 10 minutes I **Cooking time:** 10 minutes I **Servings:** 4

Ingredients:

- 2 pounds shrimp, peeled and deveined
- 1 cup cherry tomatoes, halved
- 1 tablespoon olive oil
- 4 green onion, chopped
- 1 tablespoon balsamic vinegar
- 1 tablespoon chives, chopped

Directions:

1. Heat up a pan with the oil over medium heat, add the onion, and the cherry tomatoes, stir and sauté for 4 minutes.
2. Add the shrimp and the other ingredients, cook for 6 minutes more, divide between plates and serve.

Nutrition facts per serving: calories 313, fat 7.5, fiber 1, carbs 6.4, protein 52.4

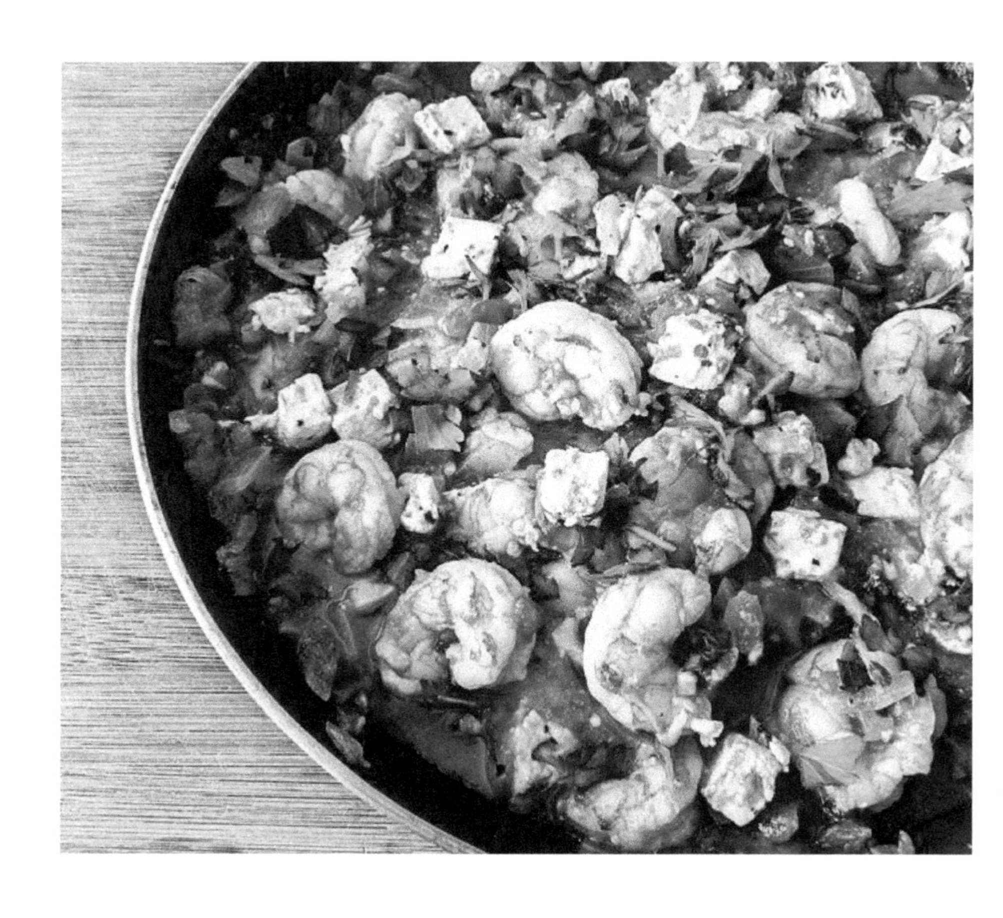

Balsamic Baby Carrots

Prep time: 10 minutes I **Cooking time:** 40 minutes I **Servings:** 4

Ingredients:

- 1 pound baby carrots, peeled
- 1 tablespoon olive oil
- 2 spring onions, chopped
- 2 tablespoons balsamic vinegar
- 2 garlic cloves, minced
- 1 teaspoon turmeric powder
- 1 tablespoon chives, chopped
- ¼ teaspoon cayenne pepper
- A pinch of salt and black pepper

Directions:

1. Spread the carrots on a baking sheet lined with parchment paper, add the oil, the spring onions and the other ingredients, toss and bake at 380 degrees F for 40 minutes.
2. Divide the carrots between plates and serve.

Nutrition facts per serving: calories 79, fat 3.8, fiber 3.7, carbs 10.9, protein 1

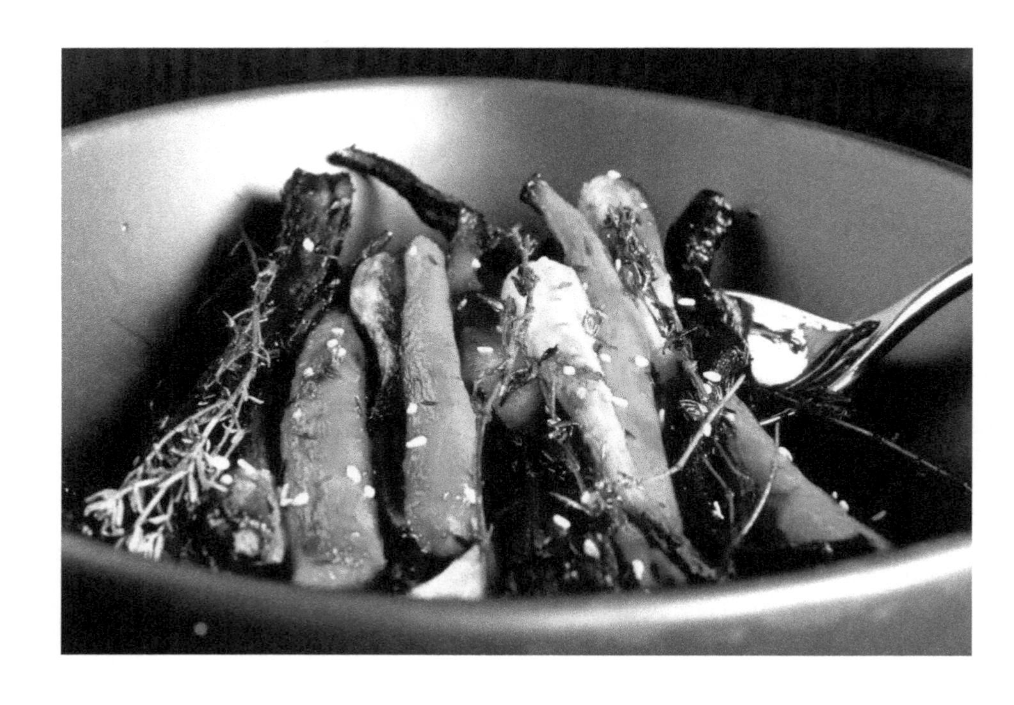

Paprika Spinach

Prep time: 10 minutes I **Cooking time:** 12 minutes I **Servings:** 4

Ingredients:

- 1 pound baby spinach
- 1 yellow onion, chopped
- 1 tablespoon olive oil
- 1 tablespoon lemon juice
- 2 garlic cloves, minced
- A pinch of cayenne pepper
- ¼ teaspoon smoked paprika
- A pinch of salt and black pepper

Directions:

1. Heat up a pan with the oil over medium-high heat, add the onion and the garlic and sauté for 2 minutes.
2. Add the spinach and the other ingredients, toss, cook over medium heat for 10 minutes, divide between plates and serve as a side dish.

Nutrition facts per serving: calories 71, fat 4, fiber 3.2, carbs 7.4, protein 3.7

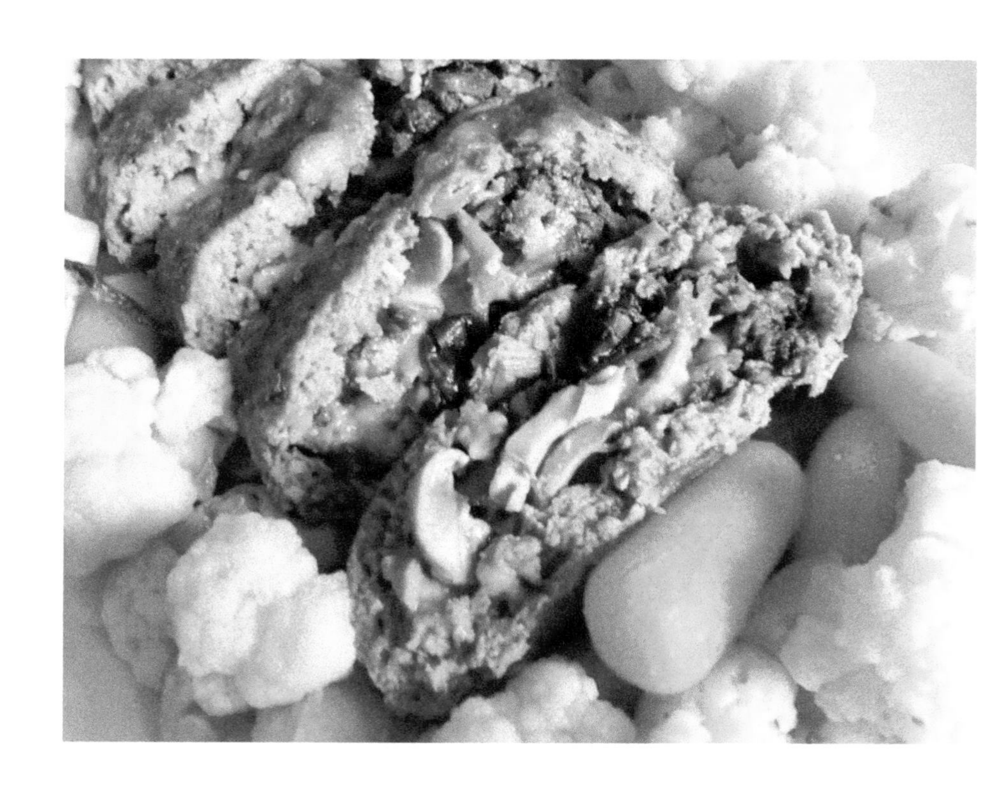

Rosemary Carrots and Onion Mix

Prep time: 5 minutes I **Cooking time:** 25 minutes I **Servings:** 4

Ingredients:

- 1 pound carrots, peeled and roughly sliced
- 1 yellow onion, chopped
- 1 tablespoon olive oil
- Zest of 1 orange, grated
- Juice of 1 orange
- 1 orange, peeled and cut into segments
- 1 tablespoon rosemary, chopped
- A pinch of salt and black pepper

Directions:

1. Heat up a pan with the oil over medium-high heat, add the onion and sauté for 5 minutes.
2. Add the carrots, the orange zest and the other ingredients, toss, cook over medium heat for 20 minutes more, divide between plates and serve.

Nutrition facts per serving: calories 140, fat 3.9, fiber 5, carbs 26.1, protein 2.1

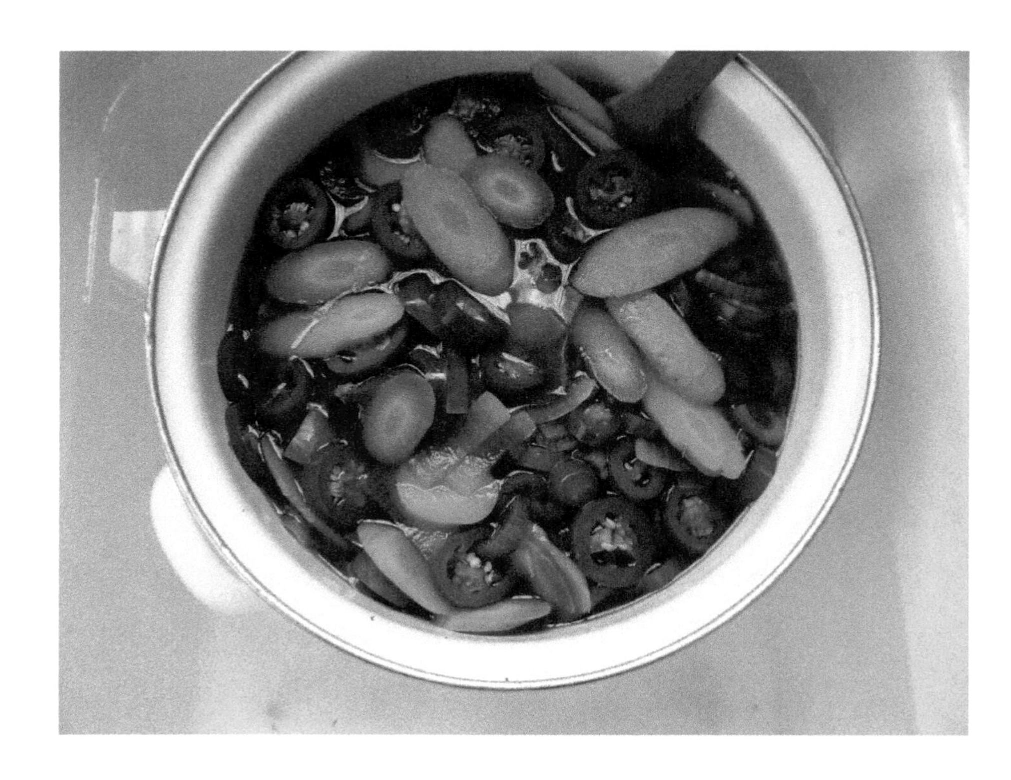

Endives and Scallions Sauté

Prep time: 5 minutes I **Cooking time:** 15 minutes I **Servings:** 4

Ingredients:

- 3 endives, shredded
- 1 tablespoon olive oil
- 4 scallions, chopped
- ½ cup tomato sauce
- 2 garlic cloves, minced
- A pinch of sea salt and black pepper
- 1/8 teaspoon turmeric powder
- 1 tablespoon chives, chopped

Directions:

1. Heat up a pan with the oil over medium heat, add the scallions and the garlic and sauté for 5 minutes.
2. Add the endives and the other ingredients, toss, cook everything for 10 minutes more, divide between plates and serve as a side dish.

Nutrition facts per serving: calories 110, fat 4.4, fiber 12.8, carbs 16.2, protein 5.6

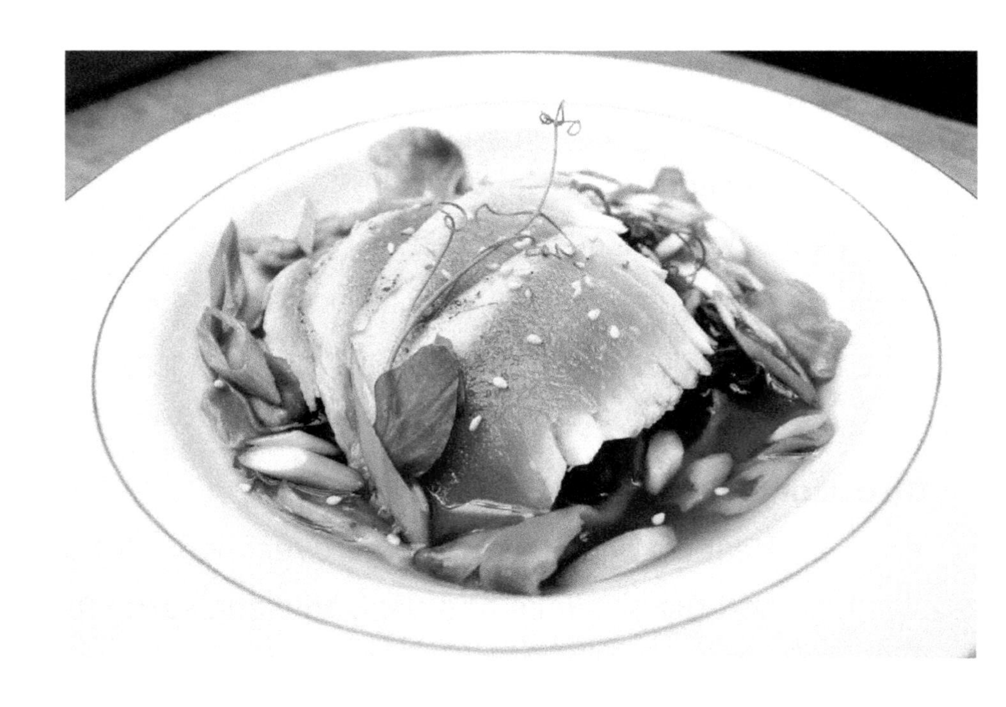

Zucchini and Apples Mix

Prep time: 5 minutes I **Cooking time:** 20 minutes I **Servings:** 4

Ingredients:

- 1 pound zucchinis, sliced
- 1 yellow onion, chopped
- 2 tablespoons olive oil
- 2 apples, peeled, cored and cubed
- 1 tomato, cubed
- 1 tablespoon rosemary, chopped
- 1 tablespoon chives, chopped

Directions:

1. Heat up a pan with the oil over medium heat, add the onion and sauté for 5 minutes.
2. Add the zucchinis and the other ingredients, toss, cook over medium heat for 15 minutes more, divide between plates and serve as a side dish.

Nutrition facts per serving: calories 170, fat 5, fiber 2, carbs 11, protein 7

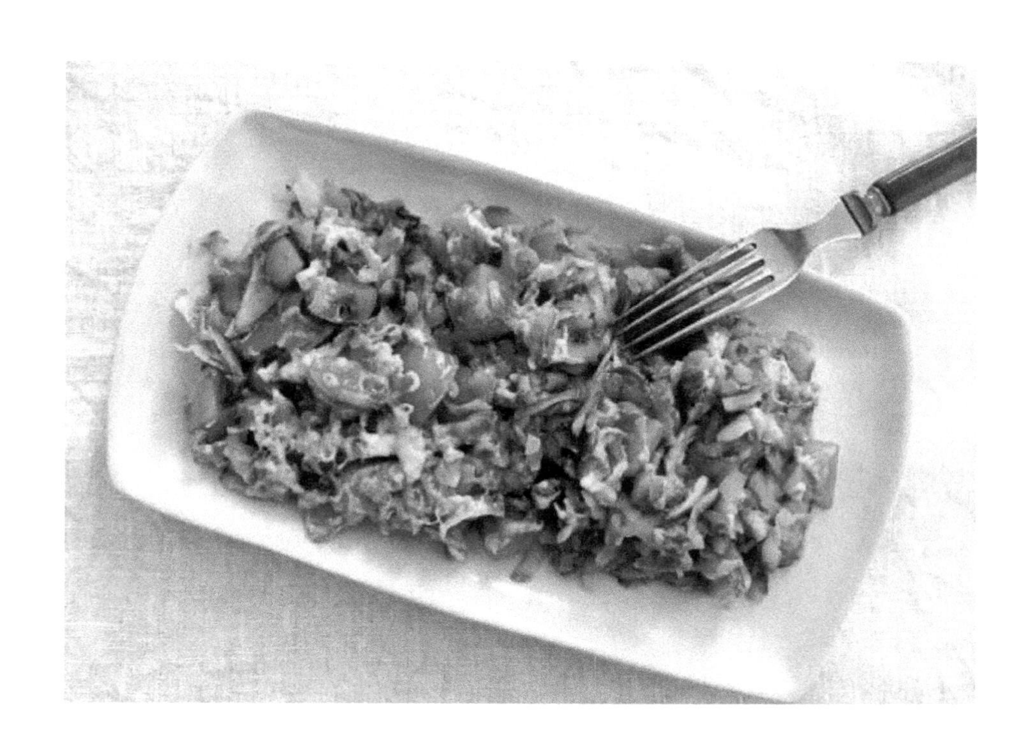

Balsamic Lime Mushrooms

Prep time: 10 minutes I **Cooking time:** 20 minutes I **Servings:** 4

Ingredients:

- 1 pound mushrooms, sliced
- 1 yellow onion, chopped
- 1 tablespoon ginger, grated
- 1 tablespoon olive oil
- 2 tablespoons balsamic vinegar
- 2 garlic cloves, minced
- A pinch of salt and black pepper
- ¼ cup lime juice
- 2 tablespoons walnuts, chopped

Directions:

1. Heat up a pan with the oil over medium-high heat, add the onion and the ginger and sauté for 5 minutes.
2. Add the mushrooms and the other ingredients, toss, cook over medium heat for 15 minutes more, divide between plates and serve.

Nutrition facts per serving: calories 120, fat 2, fiber 2, carbs 4, protein 5

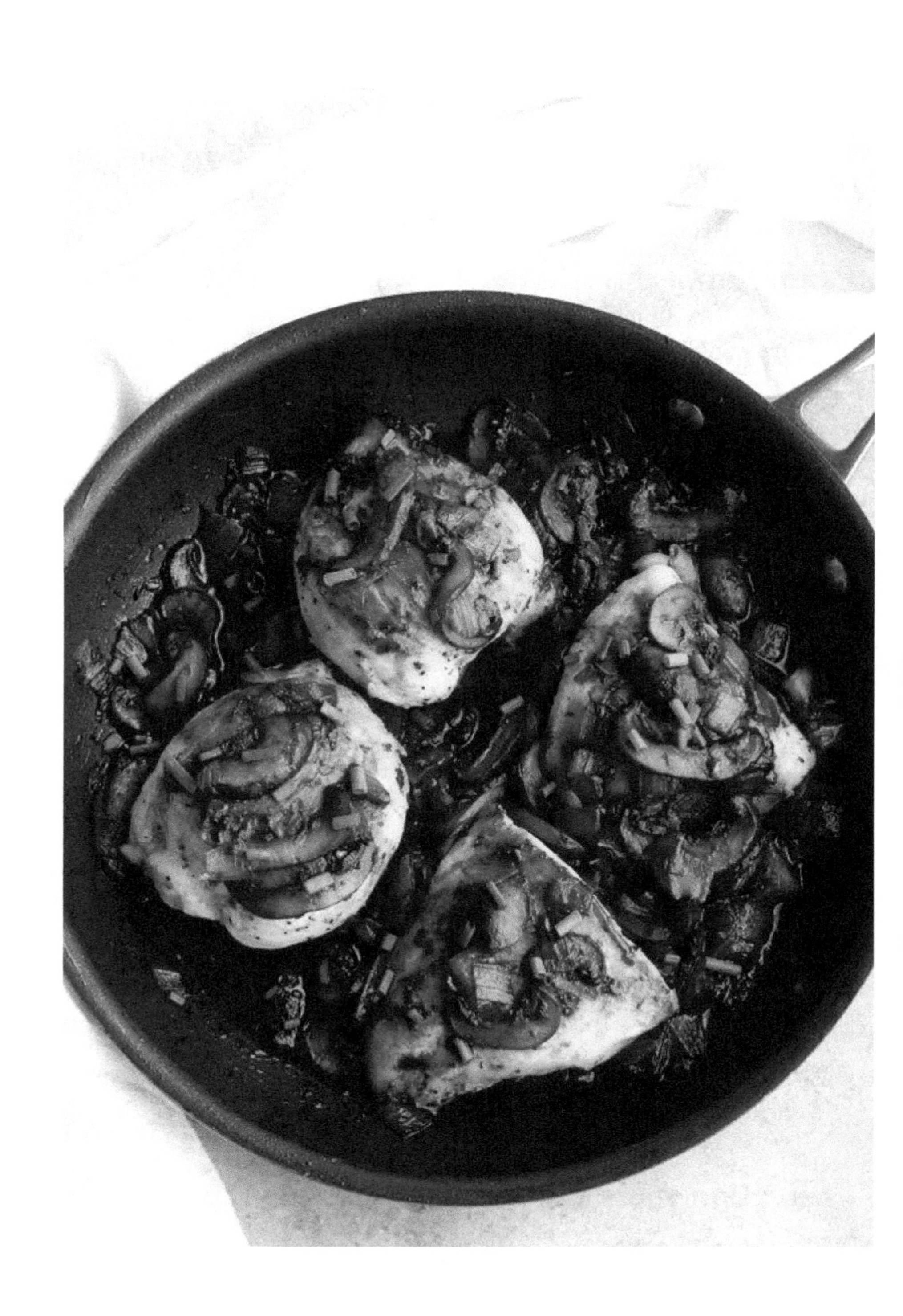

Bell Peppers and Scallions Mix

Prep time: 5 minutes I **Cooking time:** 20 minutes I **Servings:** 4

Ingredients:

- 1 red bell pepper, cut into strips
- 1 yellow bell pepper, cut into strips
- 1 green bell pepper, cut into strips
- 1 orange bell pepper, cut into strips
- 3 scallions, chopped
- 1 tablespoon olive oil
- 1 tablespoon coconut aminos
- A pinch of salt and black pepper
- 1 tablespoon parsley, chopped
- 1 tablespoon rosemary, chopped

Directions:

1. Heat up a pan with the oil over medium-high heat, add the scallions and sauté for 5 minutes.
2. Add the bell peppers and the other ingredients, toss, cook over medium heat for 15 minutes more, divide between plates and serve.

Nutrition facts per serving: calories 120, fat 1, fiber 2, carbs 7, protein 6

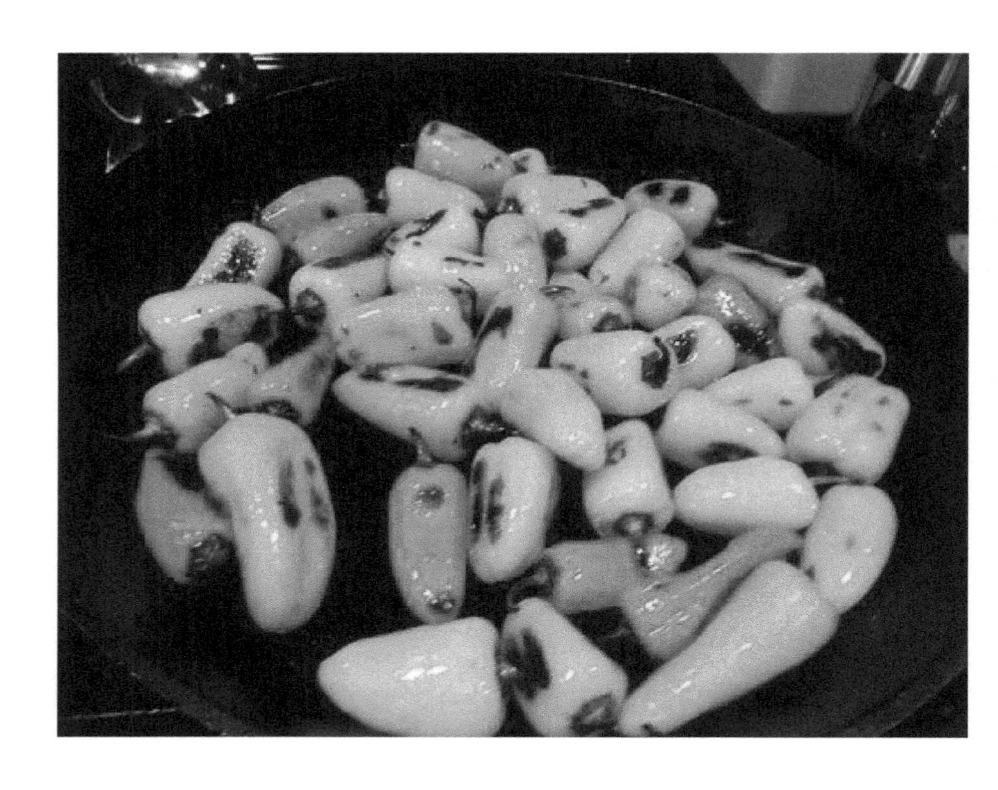

Balsamic Kale

Prep time: 5 minutes I **Cooking time:** 20 minutes I **Servings:** 4

Ingredients:

- 1 cup cherry tomatoes, halved
- 1 pound baby kale
- 1 yellow onion, chopped
- 2 tablespoons olive oil
- 1 tablespoon balsamic vinegar
- 1 tablespoon cilantro, chopped
- 2 tablespoons vegetable stock
- A pinch of salt and black pepper

Directions:

1. Heat up a pan with the oil over medium heat, add the onion and sauté for 5 minutes.
2. Add the kale, tomatoes and the other ingredients, toss, cook over medium heat for 15 minutes more, divide between plates and serve as a side dish.

Nutrition facts per serving: calories 170, fat 6, fiber 6, carbs 9, protein 4

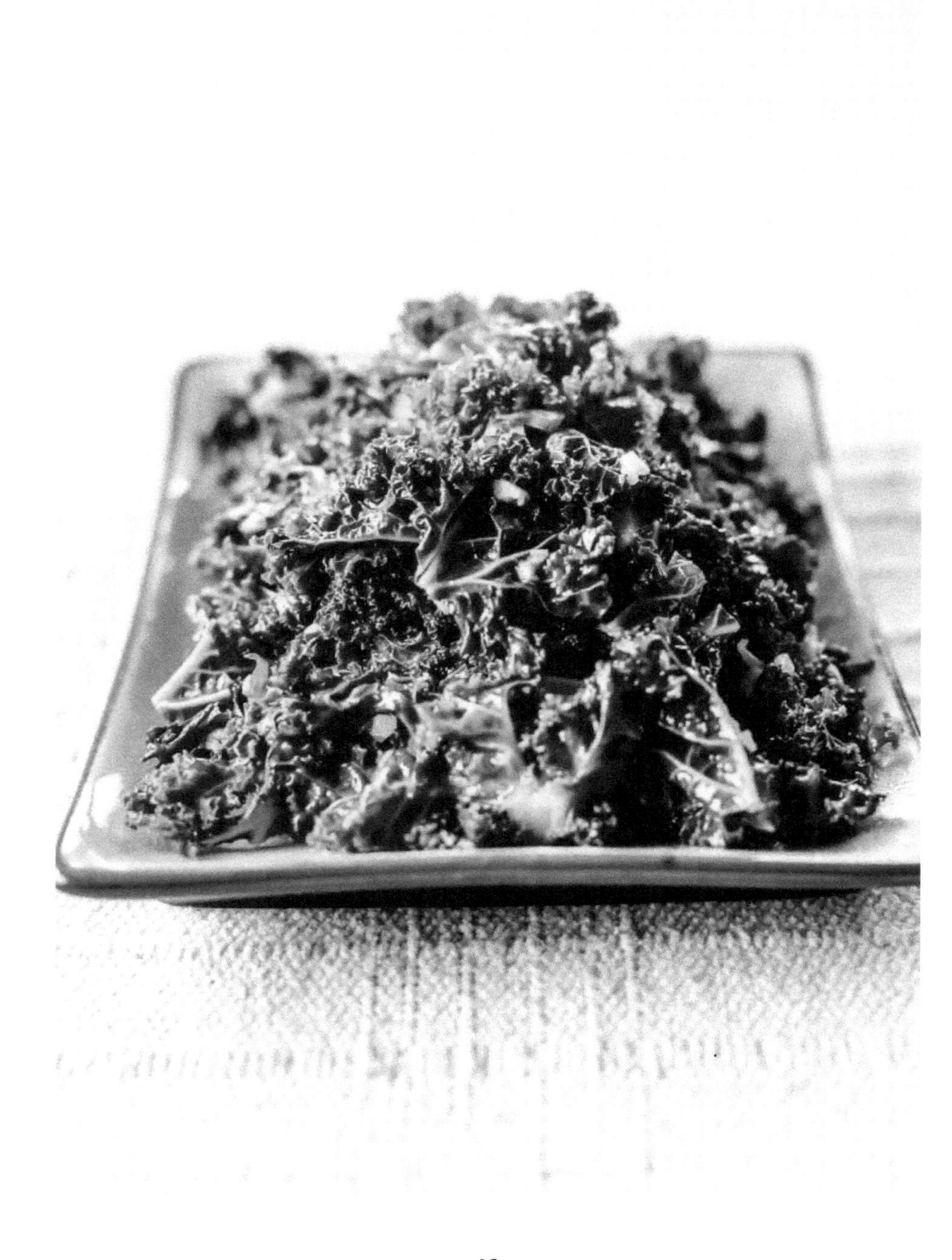

Paprika Artichokes

Prep time: 10 minutes I **Cooking time:** 25 minutes I **Servings:** 4

Ingredients:

- 2 artichokes, trimmed and halved
- 1 teaspoon chili powder
- 2 green chilies, mined
- 2 tablespoons olive oil
- 1 teaspoon garlic powder
- 1 teaspoon sweet paprika
- A pinch of salt and black pepper
- Juice of 1 lime

Directions:

1. In a roasting pan, combine the artichokes with the chili powder, the chilies and the other ingredients, toss and bake at 380 degrees F for 25 minutes.
2. Divide the artichokes between plates and serve.

Nutrition facts per serving: calories 132, fat 2, fiber 2, carbs 4, protein 6

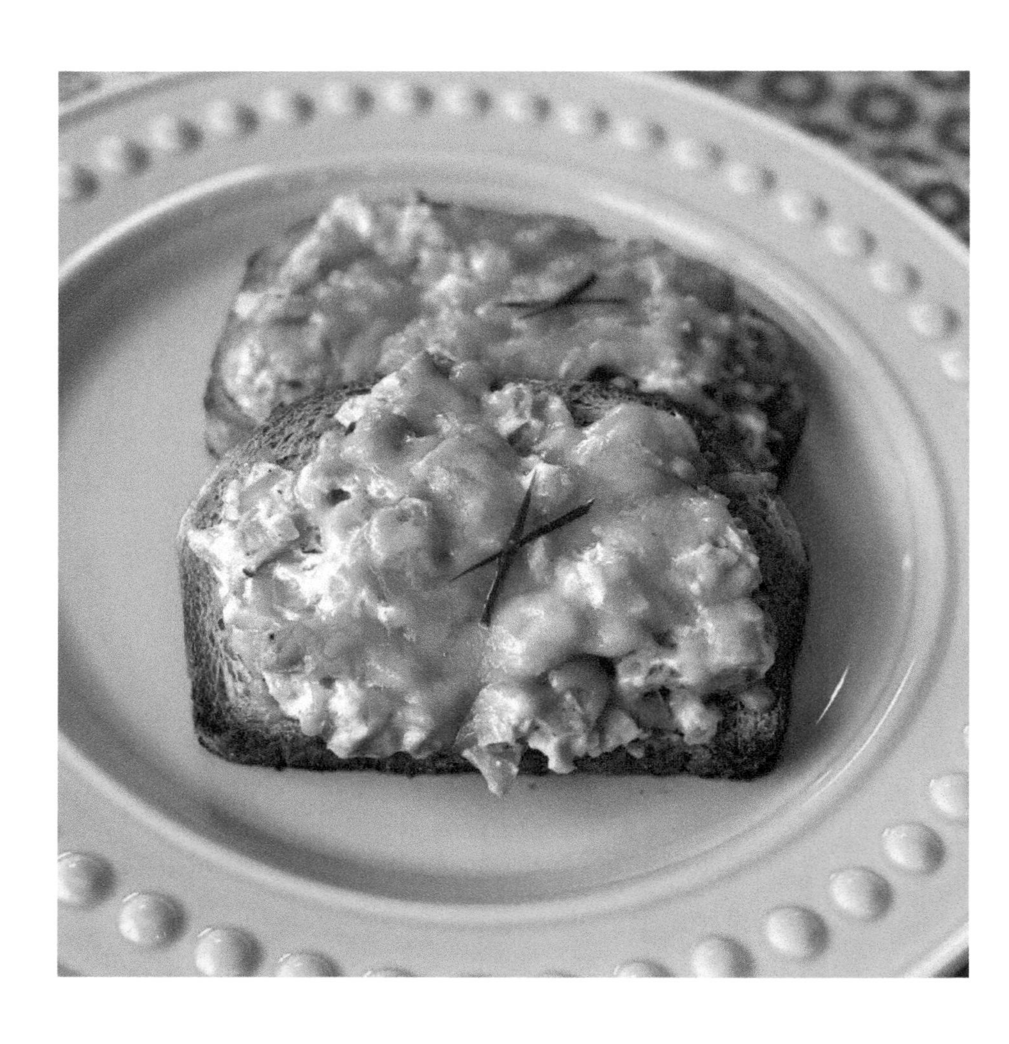

Ginger Sprouts

Prep time: 10 minutes I **Cooking time:** 20 minutes I **Servings:** 4

Ingredients:

- 2 tablespoons olive oil
- 1 pound Brussels sprouts, trimmed and halved
- 1 tablespoon ginger, grated
- 2 garlic cloves, minced
- 1 tablespoon pine nuts
- 1 tablespoon olive oil

Directions:

1. Heat up a pan with the oil over medium heat, add the garlic and the ginger and sauté for 2 minutes.
2. Add the Brussels sprouts and the other ingredients, toss, cook for 18 minutes more, divide between plates and serve.

Nutrition facts per serving: calories 160, fat 2, fiber 2, carbs 4, protein 5

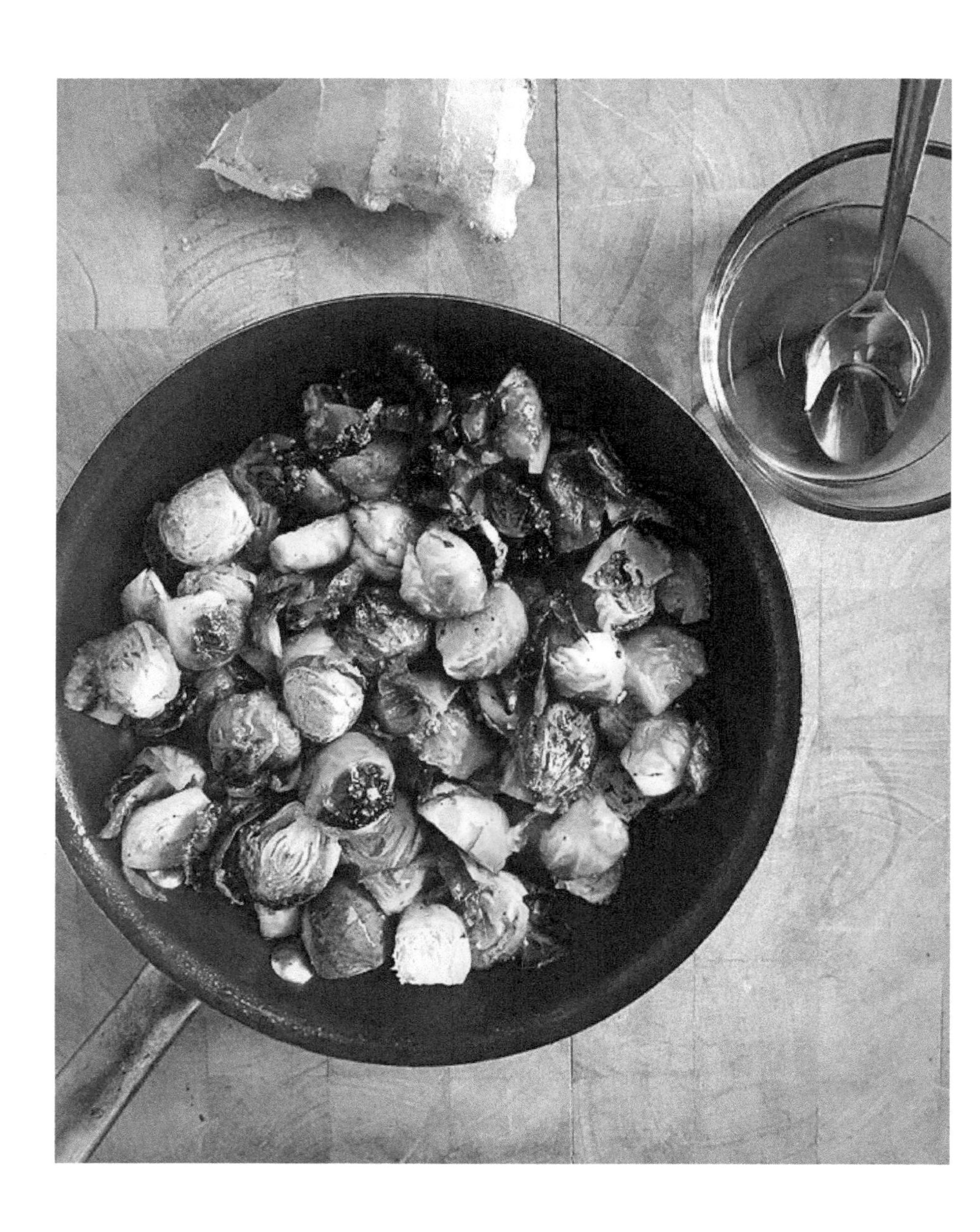

Paprika Cauliflower

Prep time: 10 minutes I **Cooking time:** 25 minutes I **Servings:** 4

Ingredients:

- 1 pound cauliflower florets
- 2 tablespoons avocado oil
- 1 teaspoon nutmeg, ground
- 1 teaspoon hot paprika
- 1 tablespoon pumpkin seeds
- 1 tablespoon chives, chopped
- A pinch of sea salt and black pepper

Directions:

1. Spread the cauliflower florets on a baking sheet lined with parchment paper, add the oil, the nutmeg and the other ingredients, toss and bake at 380 degrees F for 25 minutes.
2. Divide the cauliflower mix between plates and serve as a side dish.

Nutrition facts per serving: calories 160, fat 3, fiber 2, carbs 9, protein 4

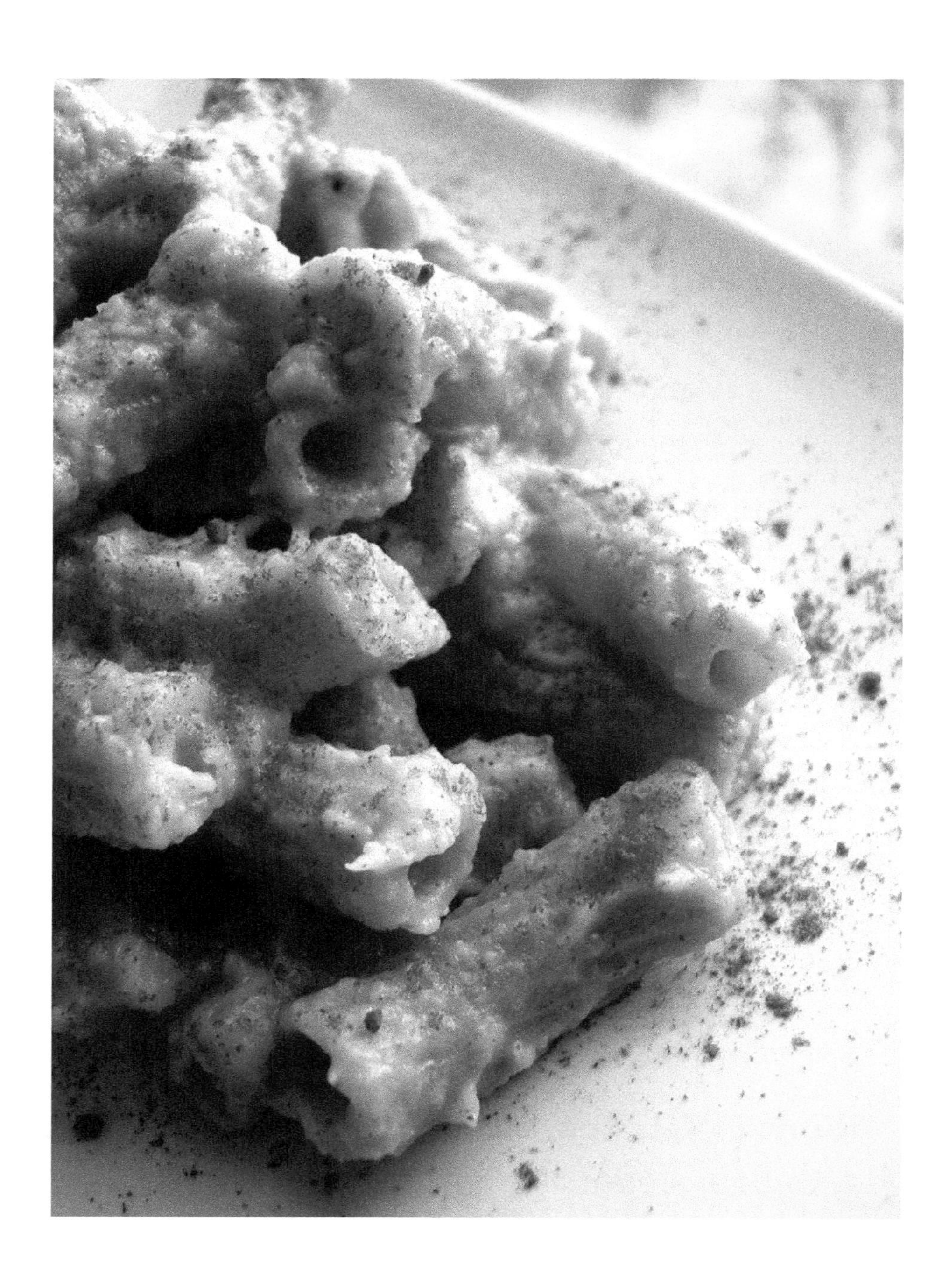

Garlic Broccoli

Prep time: 10 minutes I **Cooking time:** 30 minutes I **Servings:** 4

Ingredients:

- 2 tablespoons olive oil
- 1 pound broccoli florets
- 1 tablespoon garlic, minced
- 1 tablespoon pine nuts, toasted
- 1 tablespoon lemon juice
- 2 teaspoons mustard
- A pinch of salt and black pepper

Directions:

1. In a roasting pan, combine the broccoli with the oil, the garlic and the other ingredients, toss and bake at 380 degrees F for 30 minutes.
2. Divide everything between plates and serve as a side dish.

Nutrition facts per serving: calories 220, fat 6, fiber 2, carbs 7, protein 6

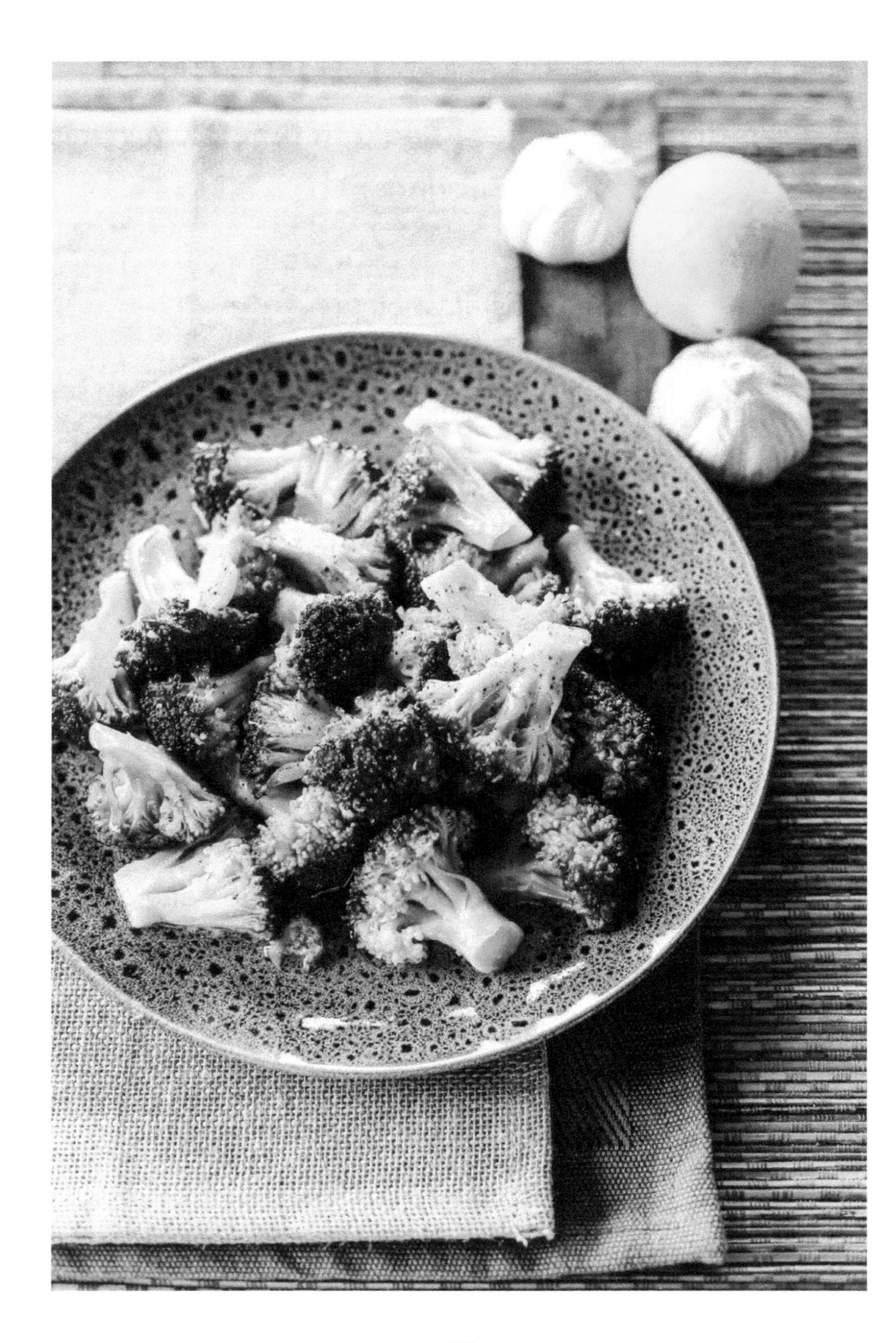

Cilantro Quinoa

Prep time: 10 minutes I **Cooking time:** 30 minutes I **Servings:** 4

Ingredients:

- 1 yellow onion, chopped
- 1 tomato, cubed
- 1 cup quinoa
- 3 cups vegetable stock
- 1 tablespoon olive oil
- 1 cup peas
- 1 tablespoon cilantro, chopped
- A pinch of salt and black pepper

Directions:

1. Heat up a pot with the oil over medium heat, add the onion, stir and sauté for 5 minutes.
2. Add the quinoa, the stock and the other ingredients, toss, bring to a simmer and cook over medium heat for 25 minutes.
3. Divide everything between plates and serve as a side dish.

Nutrition facts per serving: calories 202, fat 3, fiber 3, carbs 11, protein 6

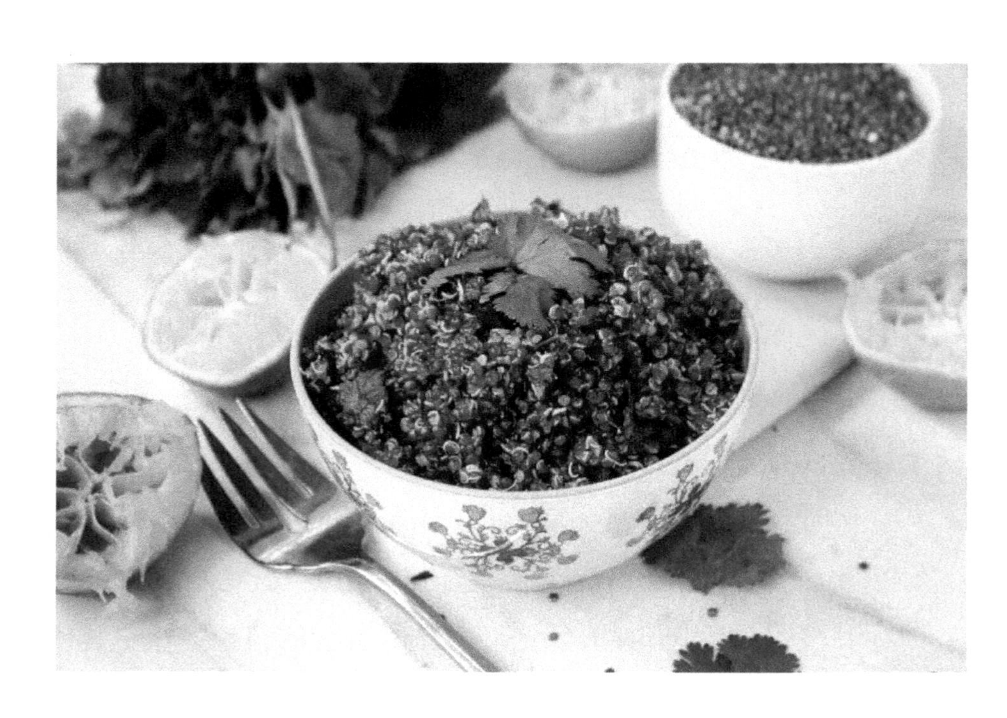

Green Beans and Sauce

Prep time: 10 minutes I **Cooking time:** 20 minutes I **Servings:** 4

Ingredients:

- 1 yellow onion, chopped
- 1 pound green beans, trimmed and halved
- 1 tablespoon avocado oil
- 2 teaspoons basil, dried
- A pinch of salt and black pepper
- 1 tablespoon tomato sauce

Directions:

1. Heat up a pan with the oil over medium-high heat, add the onion and sauté for 5 minutes.
2. Add the green beans and the other ingredients, toss, cook for 15 minutes more.
3. Divide everything between plates and serve as a side dish.

Nutrition facts per serving: calories 221, fat 5, fiber 8, carbs 10, protein 8

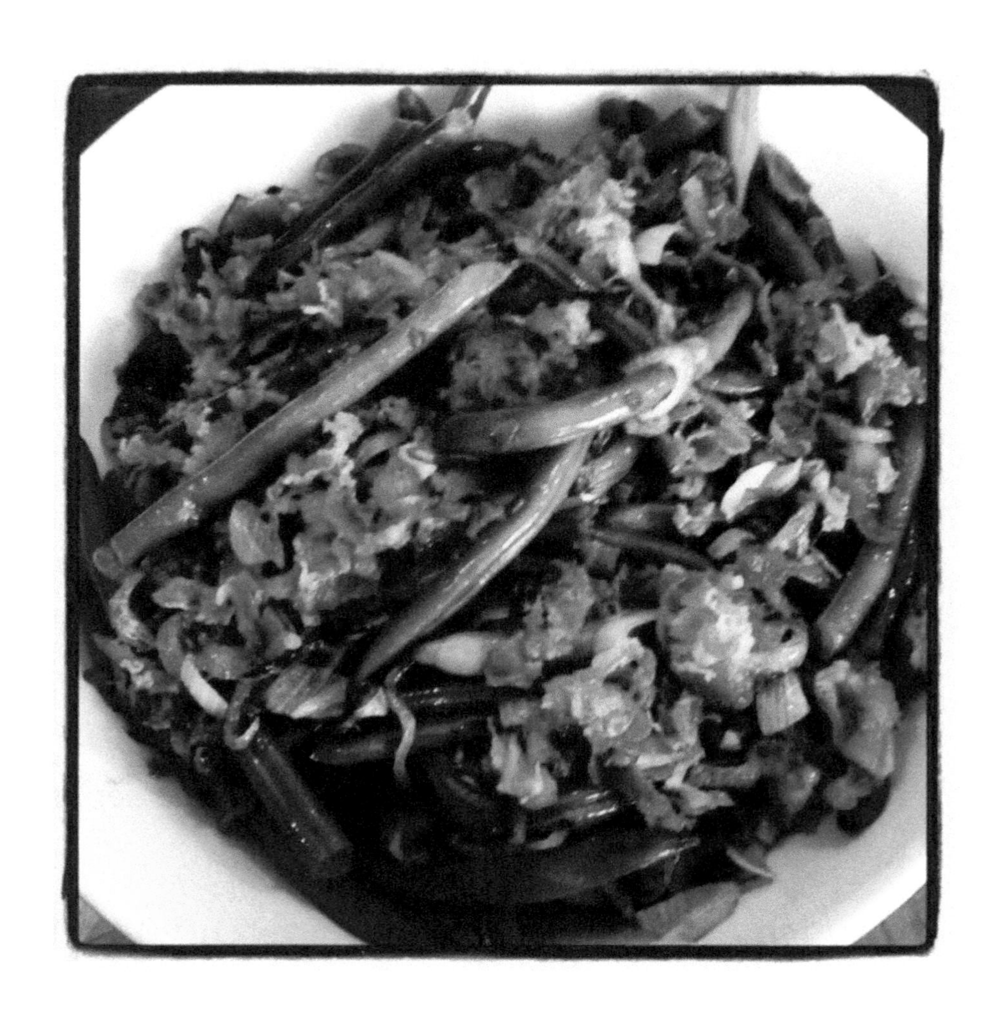

Garlic Brussels Sprouts

Prep time: 10 minutes I **Cooking time:** 20 minutes I **Servings:** 4

Ingredients:

- 2 pounds Brussels sprouts, trimmed and halved
- 1 tablespoon avocado oil
- 2 tablespoons balsamic vinegar
- 3 garlic cloves, minced
- 1 tablespoon cilantro, chopped
- A pinch of salt and black pepper

Directions:

1. Heat up a pan with the oil over medium-high heat, add the garlic and sauté for 2 minutes.
2. Add the sprouts and the other ingredients, toss, cook over medium heat for 18 minutes more, divide between plates and serve.

Nutrition facts per serving: calories 108, fat 1.2, fiber 8.7, carbs 21.7, protein 7.9

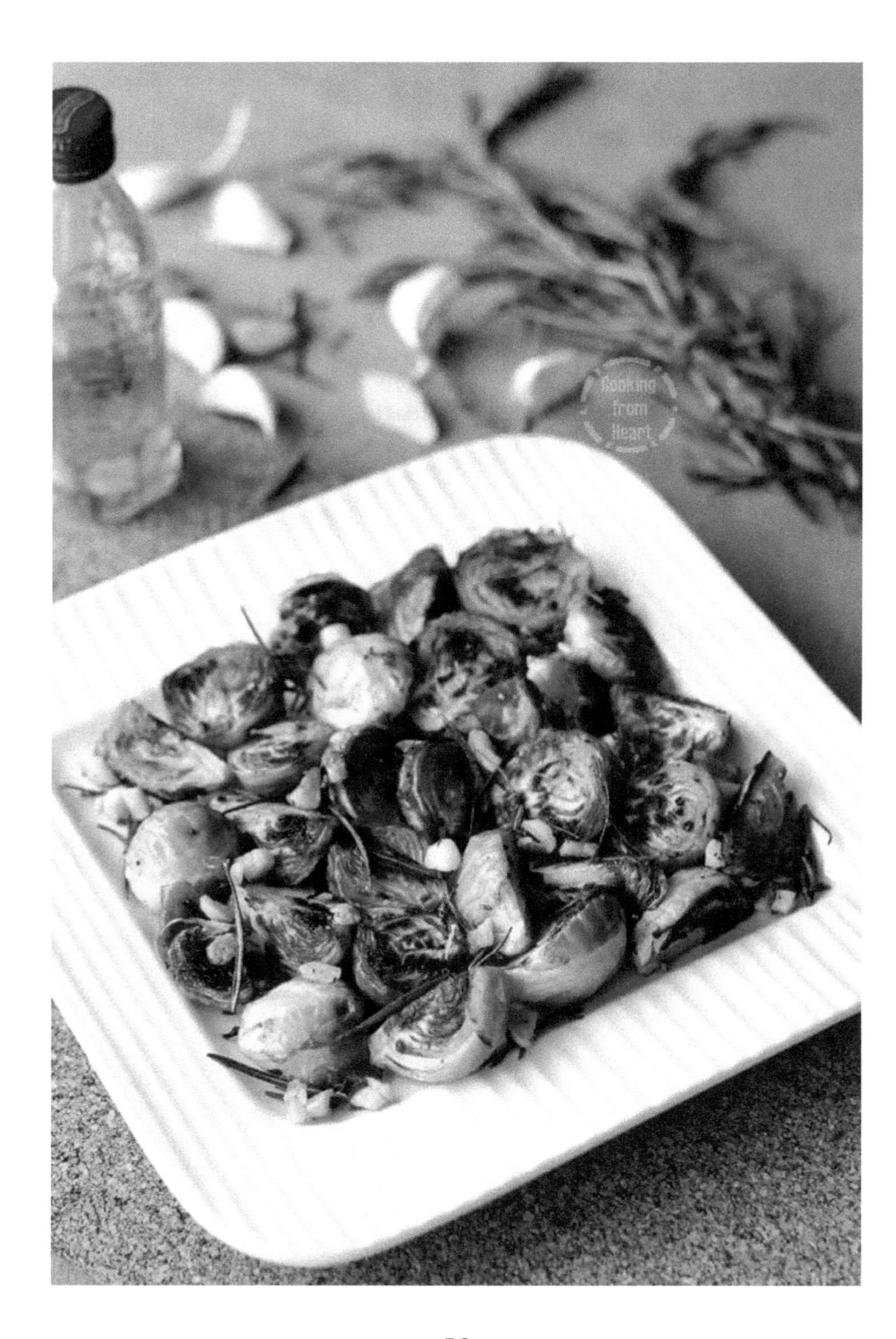
Cooking
from
Heart

Chives Cabbage

Prep time: 10 minutes I **Cooking time:** 20 minutes I **Servings:** 4

Ingredients:

- 1 green cabbage head, shredded
- 1 yellow onion, chopped
- 1 beet, peeled and cubed
- ½ cup chicken stock
- 2 tablespoons olive oil
- A pinch of salt and black pepper
- 2 tablespoons chives, chopped

Directions:

1. Heat up a pan with the oil over medium heat, add the onion and sauté for 5 minutes.
2. Add the cabbage and the other ingredients, toss, cook over medium heat for 15 minutes more, divide between plates and serve.

Nutrition facts per serving: calories 128, fat 7.3, fiber 5.6, carbs 15.6, protein 3.1

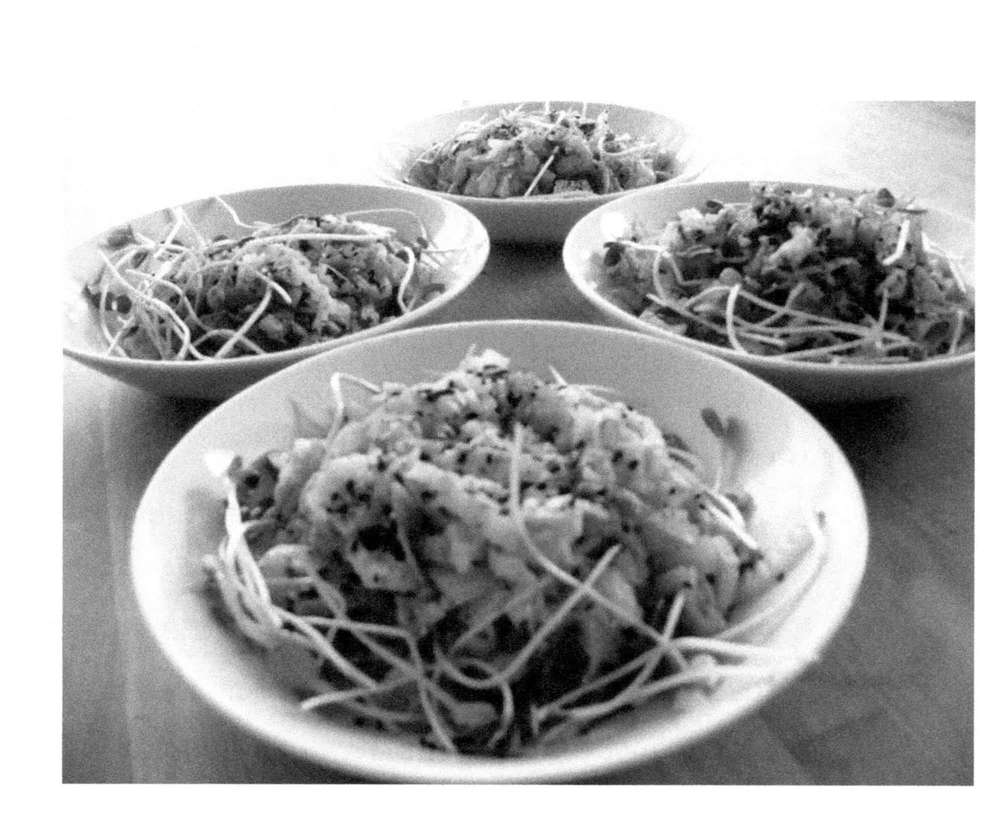

Garlic Asparagus Saute

Prep time: 10 minutes I **Cooking time:** 15 minutes I **Servings:** 4

Ingredients:

- 1 yellow onion, chopped
- 2 tablespoons olive oil
- 1 bunch asparagus, trimmed and halved
- 2 garlic cloves, minced
- 1 teaspoon chili powder
- ¼ cup cilantro, chopped

Directions:

1. Heat up a pan with the oil over medium-high heat, add the onion and the garlic and sauté for 5 minutes.
2. Add the asparagus and the other ingredients, toss, cook for 10 minutes, divide between plates and serve.

Nutrition facts per serving: calories 80, fat 7.2, fiber 1.4, carbs 4.4, protein 1

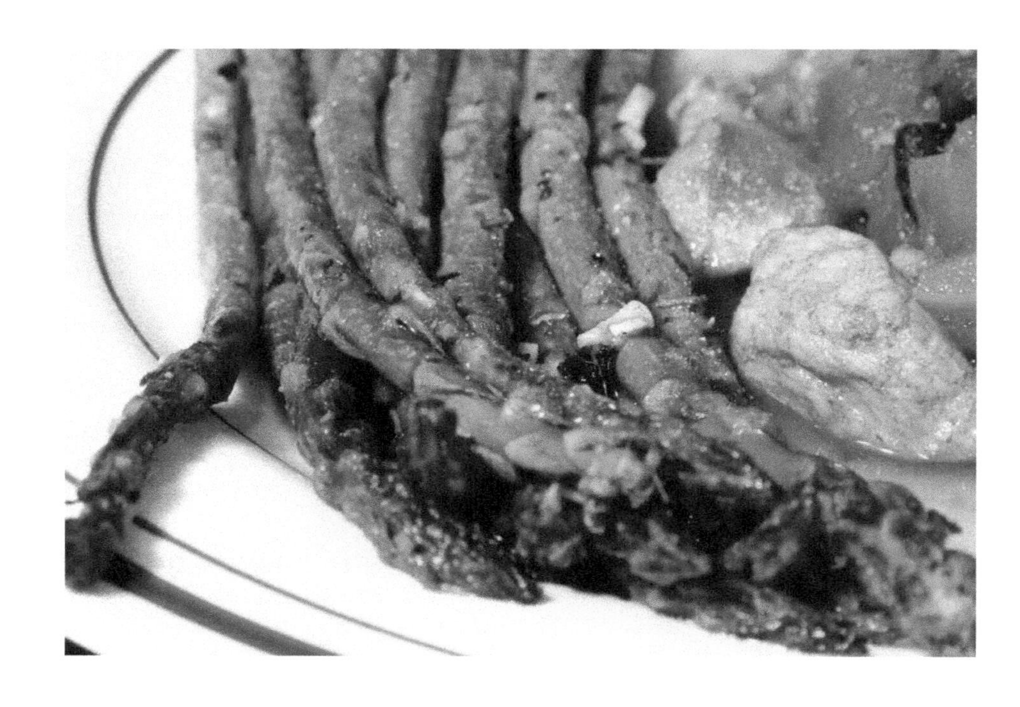

Turmeric Quinoa

Prep time: 10 minutes I **Cooking time:** 25 minutes I **Servings:** 4

Ingredients:

- 1 cup quinoa
- 3 cups chicken stock
- 1 cup tomatoes, cubed
- 1 tablespoon parsley, chopped
- 1 tablespoon basil, chopped
- 1 teaspoon turmeric powder
- A pinch of salt and black pepper

Directions:

1. In a pot, mix the quinoa with the stock, the tomatoes and the other ingredients, toss, bring to a simmer and cook over medium heat for 25 minutes.
2. Divide everything between plates and serve.

Nutrition facts per serving: calories 202, fat 4, fiber 2, carbs 12, protein 10

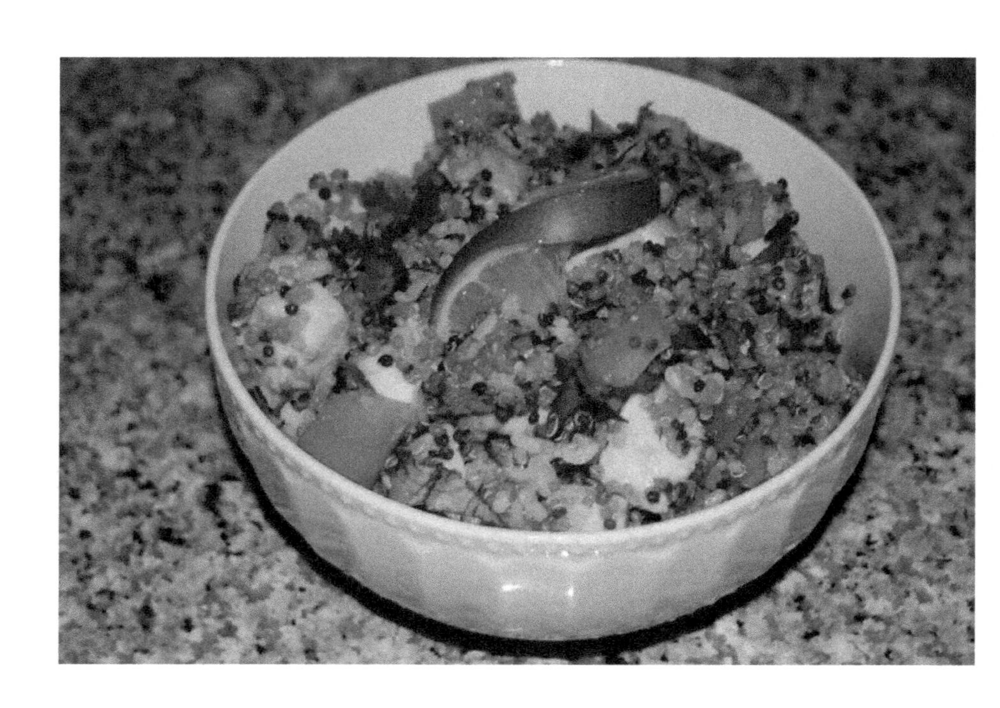

Black Beans and Peppers Mix

Prep time: 10 minutes I **Cooking time:** 20 minutes I **Servings:** 4

Ingredients:

- 1 tablespoon olive oil
- 2 cups black beans, cooked and drained
- 1 green bell pepper, chopped
- 1 yellow onion, chopped
- 4 garlic cloves, minced
- 1 teaspoon cumin, ground
- ½ cup chicken stock
- 1 tablespoon coriander, chopped
- A pinch of salt and black pepper

Directions:

1. Heat up a pan with the oil over medium heat, add the onion and the garlic and sauté for 5 minutes.
2. Add the black beans and the other ingredients, toss, cook over medium heat for 15 minutes more, divide between plates and serve.

Nutrition facts per serving: calories 221, fat 5, fiber 4, carbs 9, protein 11

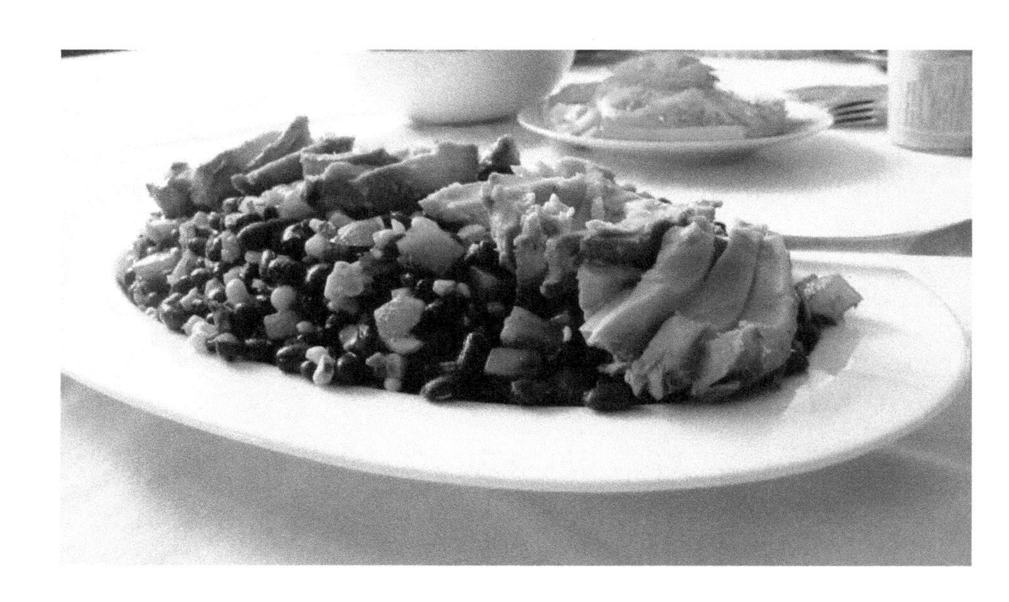

Oregano Green Beans

Prep time: 10 minutes I **Cooking time:** 20 minutes I **Servings:** 4

Ingredients:

- 1 pound green beans, trimmed and halved
- 3 scallions, chopped
- 1 mango, peeled and cubed
- 2 tablespoons olive oil
- ½ cup veggie stock
- 1 tablespoon oregano, chopped
- 1 teaspoon sweet paprika
- A pinch of salt and black pepper

Directions:

1. Heat up a pan with the oil over medium heat, add the scallions and sauté for 2 minutes.
2. Add the green beans and the other ingredients, toss, cook over medium heat for 18 minutes more, divide between plates and serve.

Nutrition facts per serving: calories 182, fat 4, fiber 5, carbs 6, protein 8

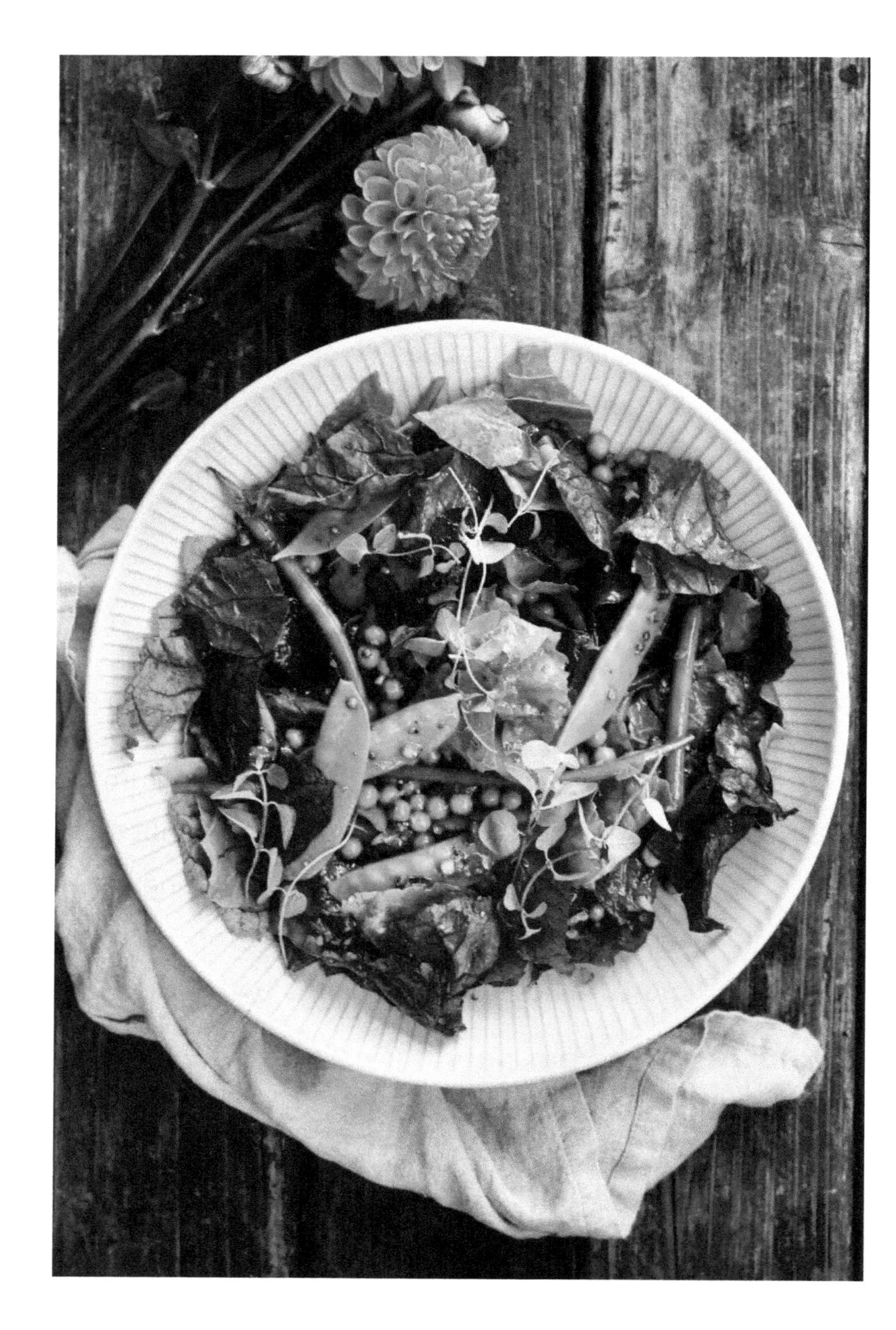

Quinoa with Green Onions

Prep time: 10 minutes I **Cooking time:** 30 minutes I **Servings:** 4

Ingredients:

- 1 yellow onion, chopped
- 1 tablespoon olive oil
- 1 cup quinoa
- 3 cups vegetable stock
- ½ cup black olives, pitted and halved
- 2 green onions, chopped
- 2 tablespoons coconut aminos
- 1 teaspoon rosemary, dried

Directions:

1. Heat up a pot with the oil over medium heat, add the yellow onion and sauté for 5 minutes.
2. Add the quinoa and the other ingredients except the green onions, stir, bring to a simmer and cook over medium heat for 25 minutes.
3. Divide the mix between plates, sprinkle the green onions on top and serve.

Nutrition facts per serving: calories 261, fat 6, fiber 8, carbs 10, protein 6

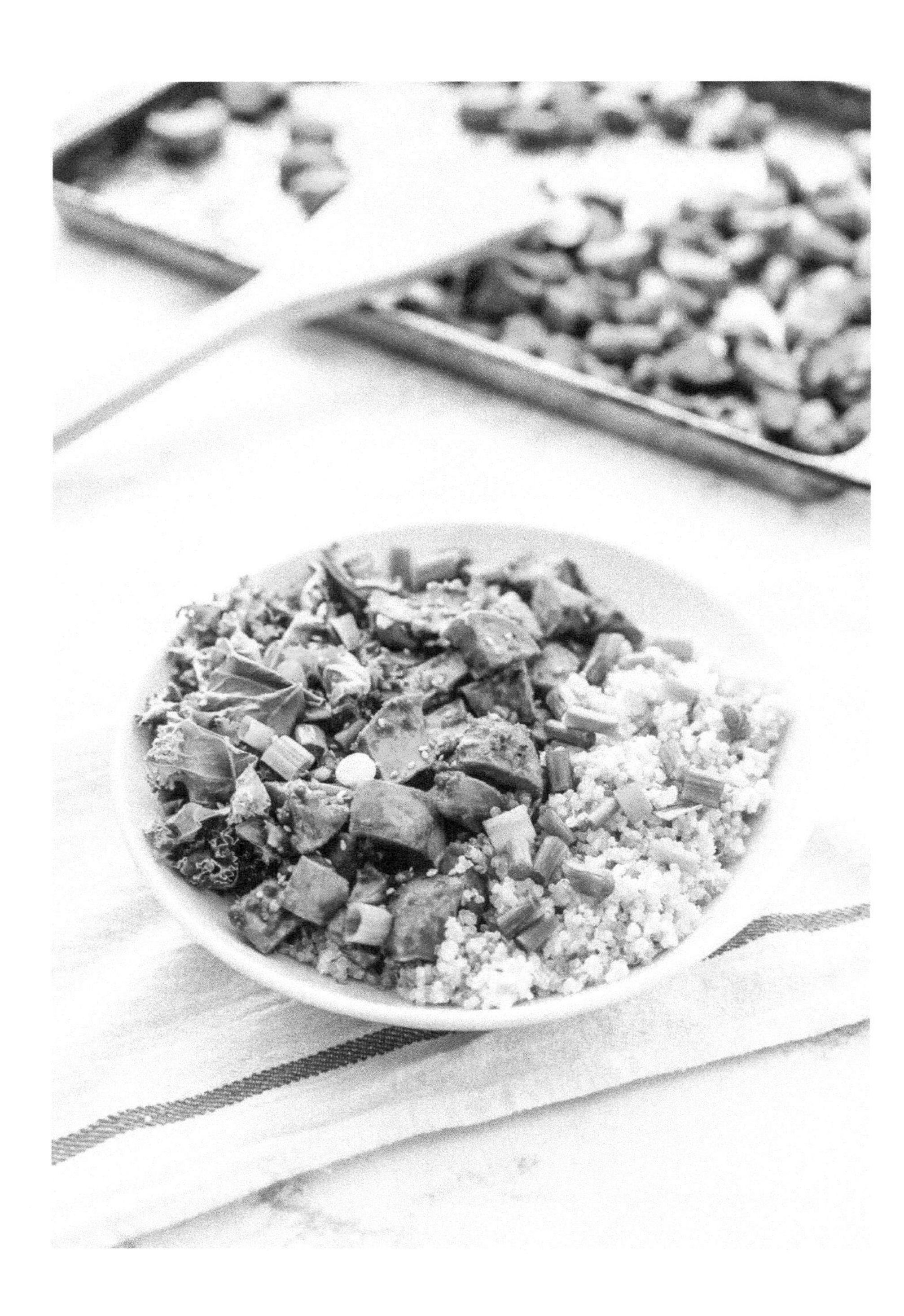

Dill Zucchini Cream

Prep time: 10 minutes I **Cooking time:** 20 minutes I **Servings:** 4

Ingredients:

- 1 tablespoon olive oil
- 1 yellow onion, chopped
- 1 teaspoon ginger, grated
- 1 pound zucchinis, chopped
- 32 ounces chicken stock
- 1 cup coconut cream
- 1 tablespoon dill, chopped

Directions:

1. Heat up a pot with the oil over medium heat, add the onion and ginger, stir and cook for 5 minutes.
2. Add the zucchinis and the other ingredients, bring to a simmer and cook over medium heat for 15 minutes.
3. Blend using an immersion blender, divide into bowls and serve.

Nutrition facts per serving: calories 293, fat 12.3, fiber 2.7, carbs 11.2, protein 6.4

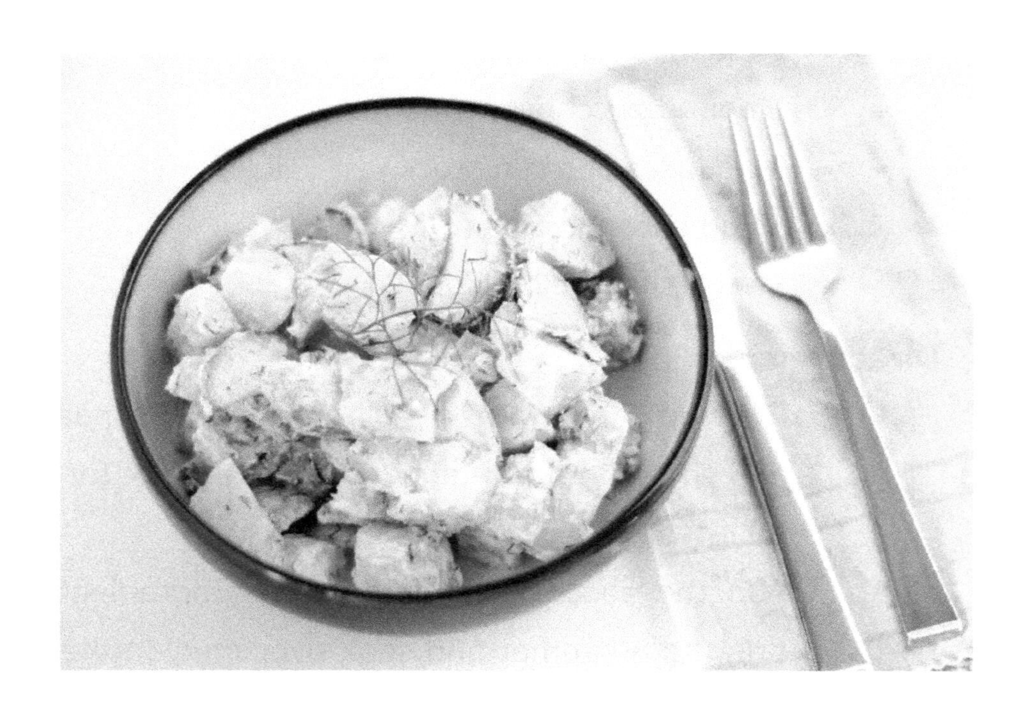

Shrimp, Walnuts and Grapes Bowls

Prep time: 5 minutes I **Cooking time:** 0 minutes I **Servings:** 4

Ingredients:

- 2 tablespoons mayonnaise
- 2 teaspoons chili powder
- A pinch of black pepper
- 1 pound shrimp, cooked, peeled and deveined
- 1 cup red grapes, halved
- ½ cup scallions, chopped
- ¼ cup walnuts, chopped
- 1 tablespoon cilantro, chopped

Directions:

1. In a salad bowl, combine shrimp with the chili powder and the other ingredients, toss and serve fro lunch.

Nutrition facts per serving: calories 298, fat 12.3, fiber 2.6, carbs 16.2, protein 7.8

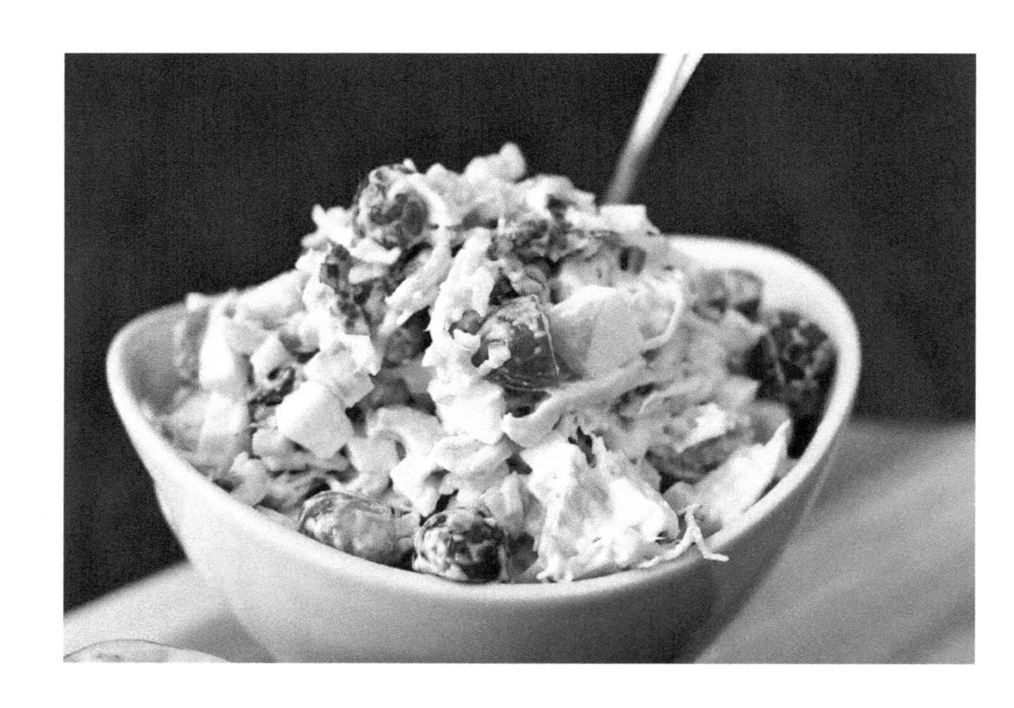

Carrot and Celery Cream

Prep time: 5 minutes I **Cooking time:** 25 minutes I **Servings:** 4

Ingredients:

- 2 tablespoons olive oil
- 1 yellow onion, chopped
- 1 pound carrots, peeled and chopped
- 1 teaspoon turmeric powder
- 4 celery stalks, chopped
- 5 cups chicken stock
- A pinch of black pepper
- 1 tablespoon cilantro, chopped

Directions:

1. Heat up a pot with the oil over medium heat, add the onion, stir and sauté for 2 minutes.
2. Add the carrots and the other ingredients, bring to a simmer and cook over medium heat for 20 minutes.
3. Blend the soup using an immersion blender, ladle into bowls and serve.

Nutrition facts per serving: calories 221, fat 9.6, fiber 4.7, carbs 16, protein 4.8

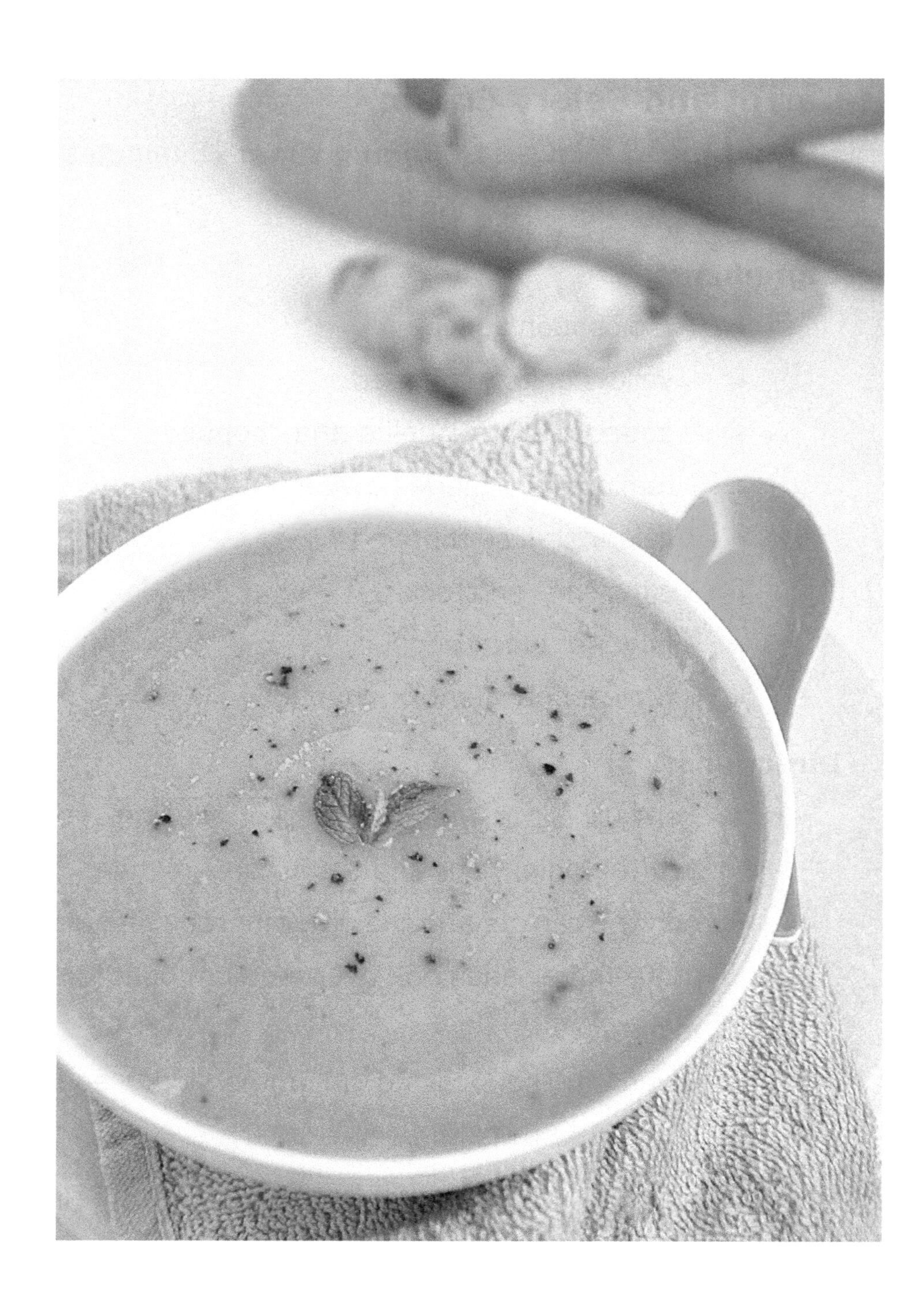

Beef Soup

Prep time: 10 minutes I **Cooking time:** 1 hour and 40 minutes I **Servings:** 4

Ingredients:

- 1 cup black beans, cooked
- 7 cups beef stock
- 1 green bell pepper, chopped
- 1 tablespoon olive oil
- 1 pound beef stew meat, cubed
- 1 yellow onion, chopped
- 3 garlic cloves, minced
- 1 chili pepper, chopped
- 1 potato, cubed
- A pinch of black pepper
- 1 tablespoon cilantro, chopped

Directions:

1. Heat up a pot with the oil over medium heat, add the onion, garlic and the meat, and brown for 5 minutes.
2. Add the beans and the rest of the ingredients except the cilantro, bring to a simmer and cook over medium heat for 1 hour and 35 minutes.
3. Add the cilantro, ladle the soup into bowls and serve.

Nutrition facts per serving: calories 421, fat 17.3, fiber 3.8, carbs 18.8, protein 23.5

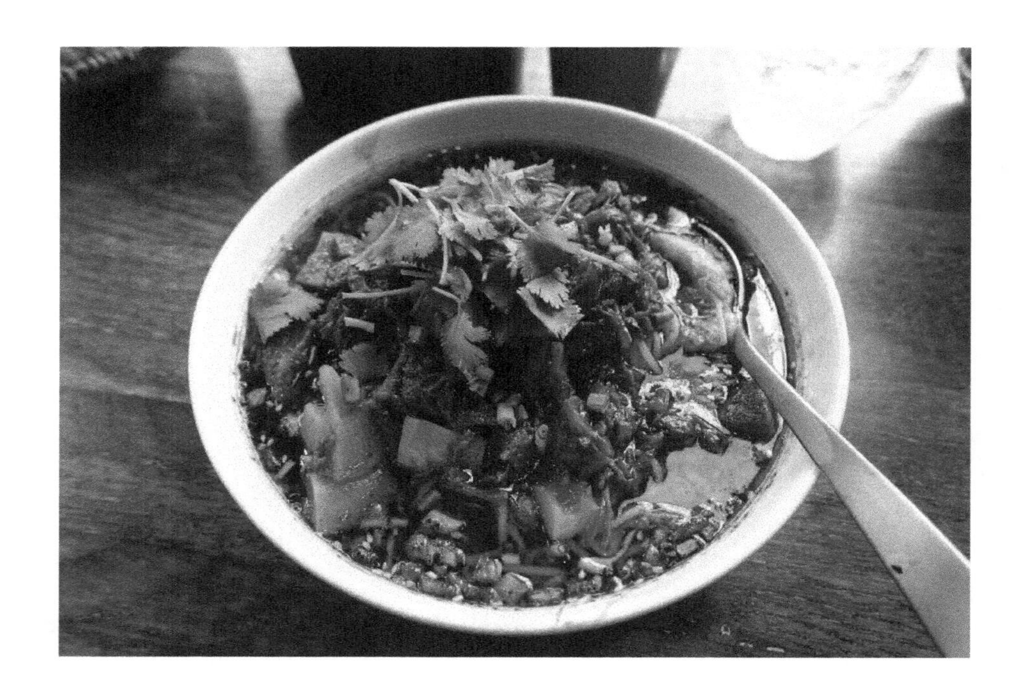

Salmon and Salsa Bowls

Prep time: 10 minutes I **Cooking time:** 13 minutes I **Servings:** 4

Ingredients:

- ½ pound smoked salmon, boneless, skinless and cubed
- ½ pound shrimp, peeled and deveined
- 1 tablespoon olive oil
- 1 red onion, chopped
- ¼ cup tomatoes, cubed
- ½ cup mild salsa
- 2 tablespoons cilantro, chopped

Directions:

1. Heat up a pan with the oil over medium-high heat, add the salmon, toss and cook for 5 minutes.
2. Add the onion, shrimp and the other ingredients, cook for 7 minutes more, divide into bowls and serve.

Nutrition facts per serving: calories 251, fat 11.4, fiber 3.7, carbs 12.3, protein 7.1

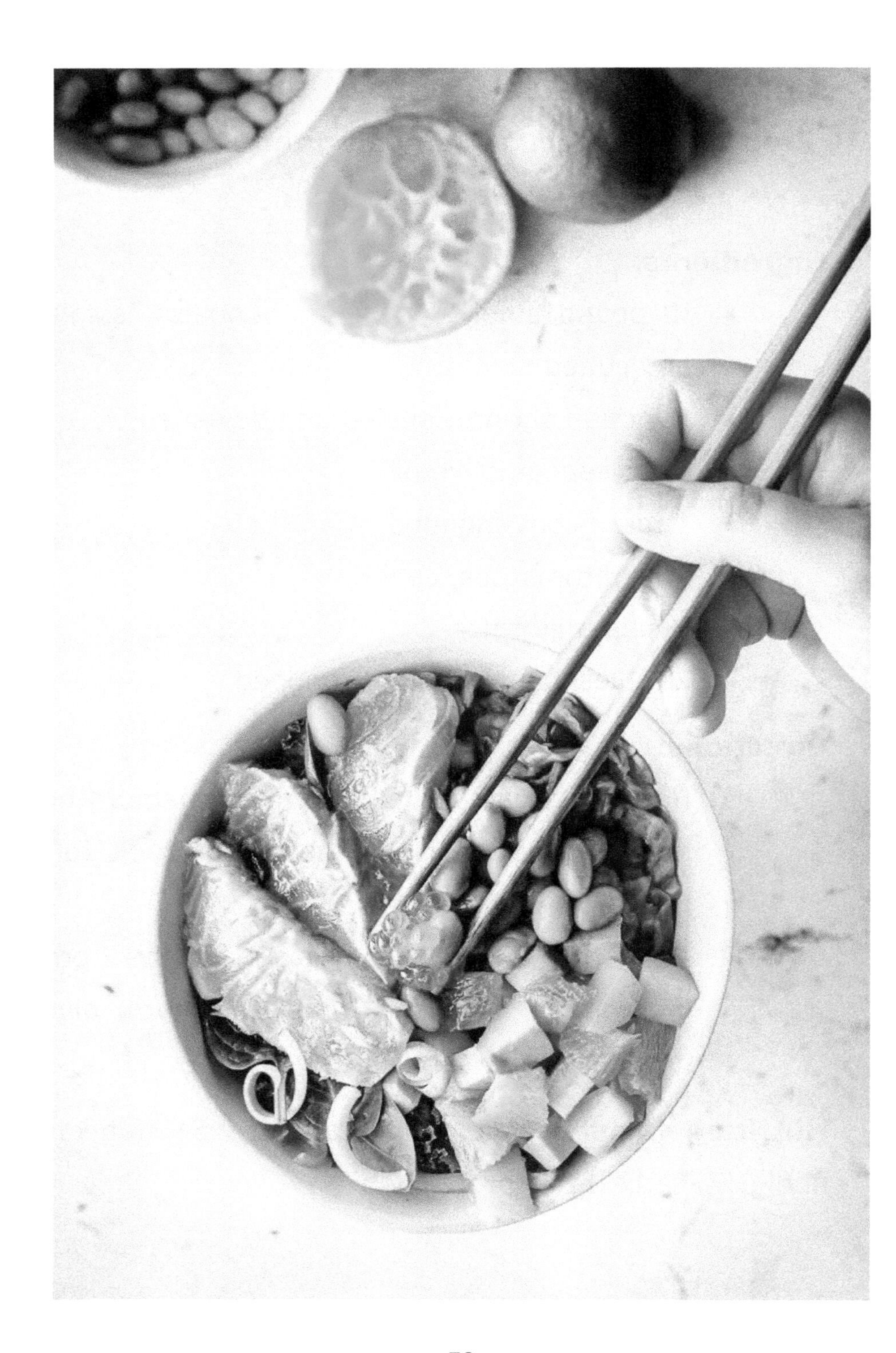

Chicken and Herbs Sauce

Prep time: 5 minutes I **Cooking time:** 20 minutes I **Servings:** 4

Ingredients:

- 1 tablespoon olive oil
- 1 yellow onion, chopped
- A pinch of black pepper
- 1 pound chicken breasts, skinless, boneless and cubed
- 4 garlic cloves, minced
- 1 cup chicken stock
- 2 cups coconut cream
- 1 tablespoon basil, chopped
- 1 tablespoon chives, chopped

Directions:

1. Heat up a pan with the oil over medium-high heat, add the garlic, onion and the meat, toss and brown for 5 minutes.
2. Add the stock and the rest of the ingredients, bring to a simmer and cook over medium heat for 15 minutes.
3. Divide the mix between plates and serve.

Nutrition facts per serving: calories 451, fat 16.6, fiber 9, carbs 34.4, protein 34.5

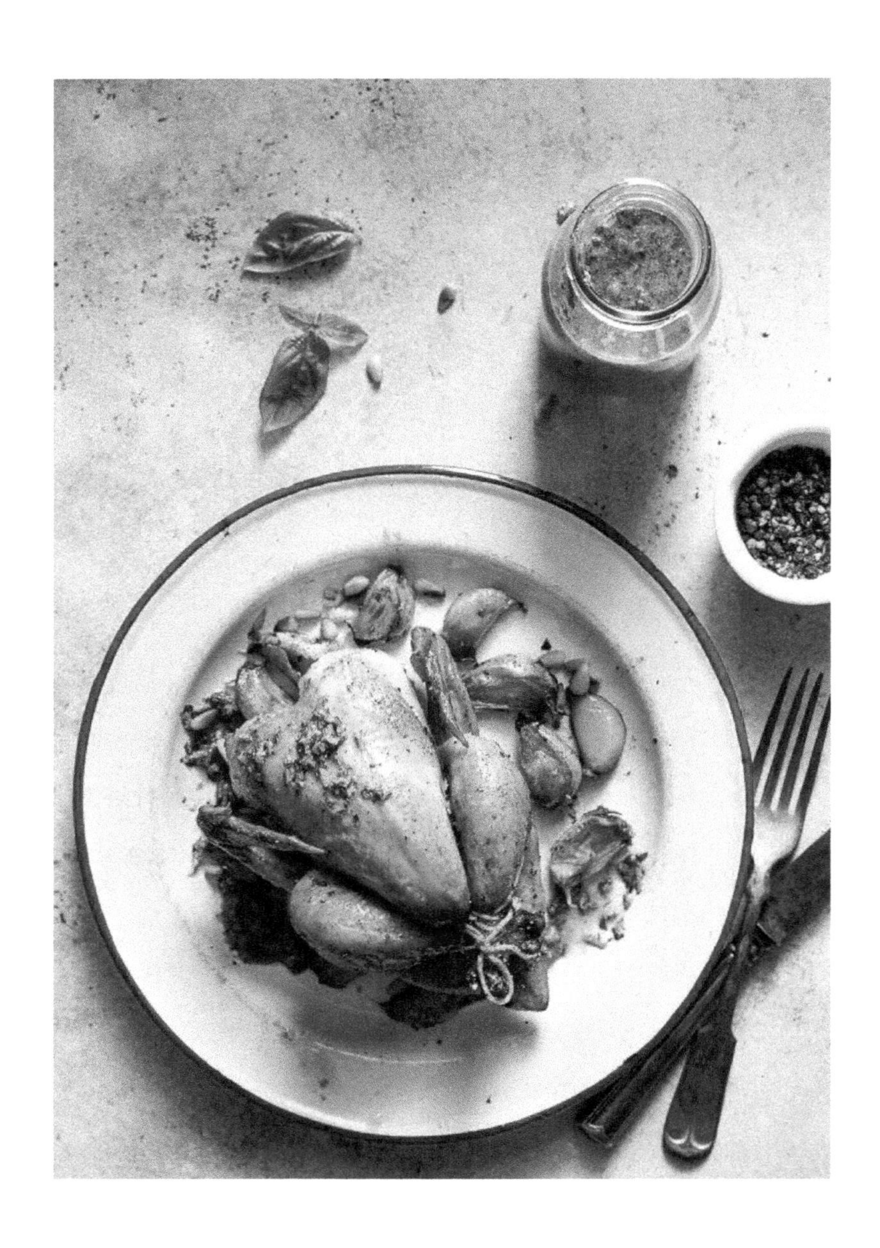

Ginger Chicken and Veggies Stew

Prep time: 5 minutes I **Cooking time:** 20 minutes I **Servings:** 4

Ingredients:

- 1 pound chicken breasts, skinless, boneless and cubed
- 2 shallots, chopped
- 1 tablespoon olive oil
- 1 eggplant, cubed
- 1 cup tomatoes, crushed
- 1 tablespoon lime juice
- A pinch of black pepper
- ¼ teaspoon ginger, ground
- 1 tablespoon cilantro, chopped

Directions:

1. Heat up a pot with the oil over medium heat, add the shallots and the chicken and brown for 5 minutes.
2. Add the rest of the ingredients, bring to a simmer and cook over medium heat for 15 minutes more.
3. Divide into bowls and serve for lunch.

Nutrition facts per serving: calories 441, fat 14.6, fiber 4.9, carbs 44.4, protein 16.9

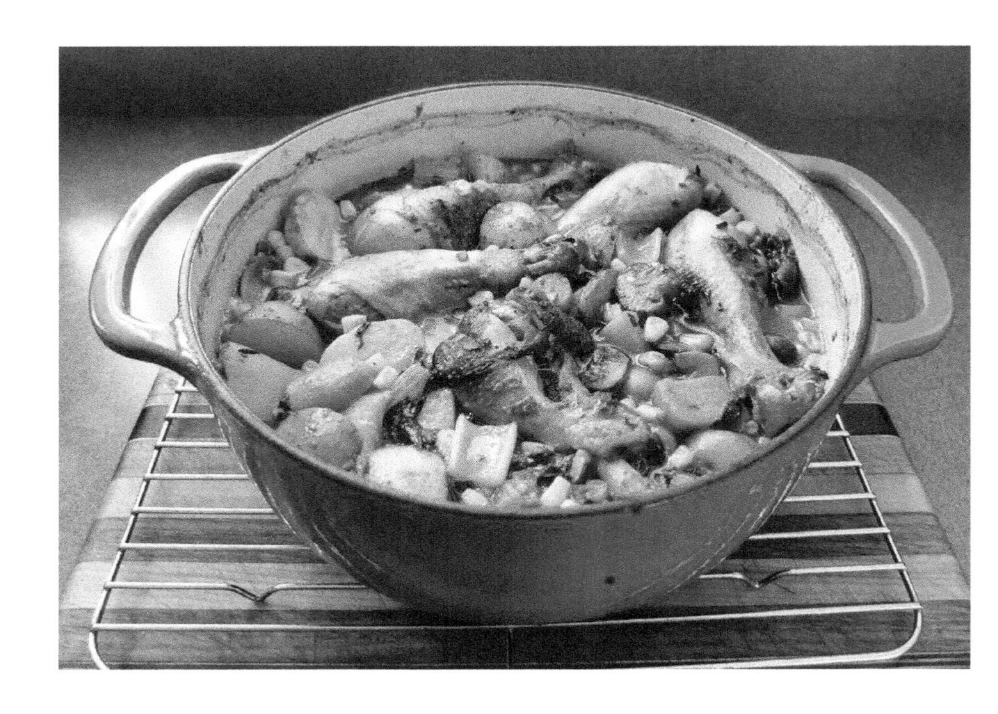

Chives Chicken and Endives

Prep time: 5 minutes I **Cooking time:** 20 minutes I **Servings:** 4

Ingredients:

- 1 pound chicken thighs, boneless, skinless and cubed
- 2 endives, shredded
- 1 cup chicken stock
- 1 tablespoon olive oil
- 1 yellow onion, chopped
- 1 carrot, sliced
- 2 garlic cloves, minced
- 8 ounces tomatoes, chopped
- 1 tablespoon chives, chopped

Directions:

1. Heat up a pan with the oil over medium-high heat, add the onion and garlic and sauté for 5 minutes.
2. Add the chicken and brown for 5 minutes more.
3. Add the rest of the ingredients, bring to a simmer, cook for 10 minutes more, divide between plates and serve.

Nutrition facts per serving: calories 411, fat 16.7, fiber 5.9, carbs 54.5, protein 24

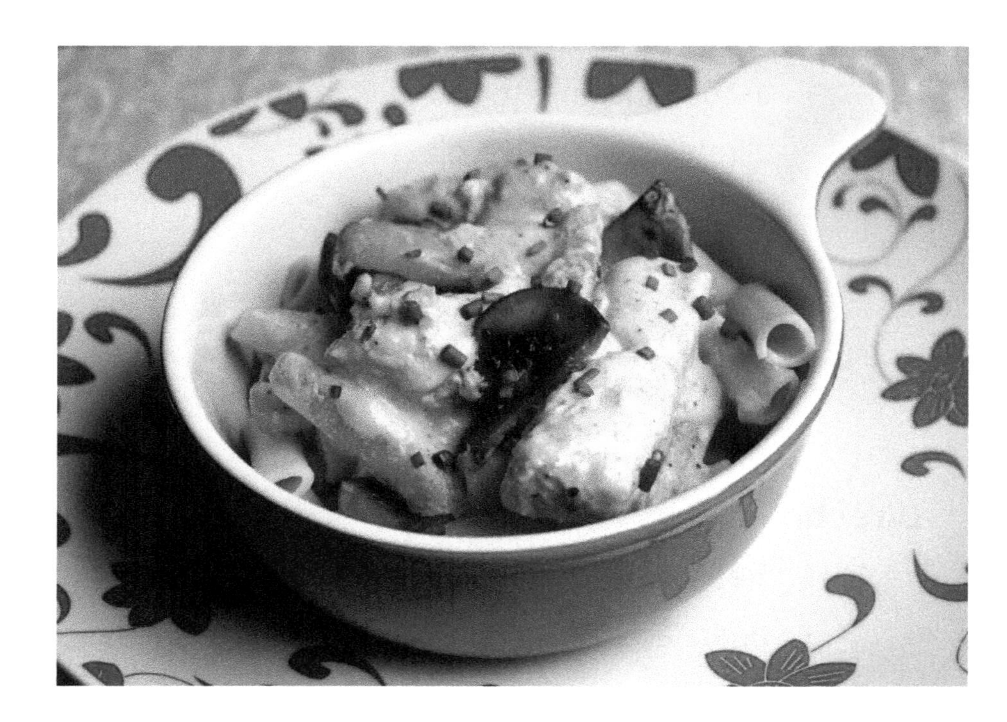

Oregano Turkey and Garlic Soup

Prep time: 10 minutes I **Cooking time:** 40 minutes I **Servings:** 4

Ingredients:

- 1 turkey breast, skinless, boneless, cubed
- 1 tablespoon tomato paste
- 1 tablespoon olive oil
- 2 yellow onions, chopped
- 1 quart chicken stock
- 1 tablespoon oregano, chopped
- 2 carrots, sliced
- 3 garlic cloves, minced
- A pinch of black pepper

Directions:

1. Heat up a pot with the oil over medium heat, add the onions and the garlic and sauté for 5 minutes.
2. Add the meat and brown it for 5 minutes more.
3. Add the rest of the ingredients, bring to a simmer and cook over medium heat for 30 minutes.
4. Ladle the soup into bowls and serve.

Nutrition facts per serving: calories 321, fat 14.5, fiber 11.3, carbs 33.7, protein 16

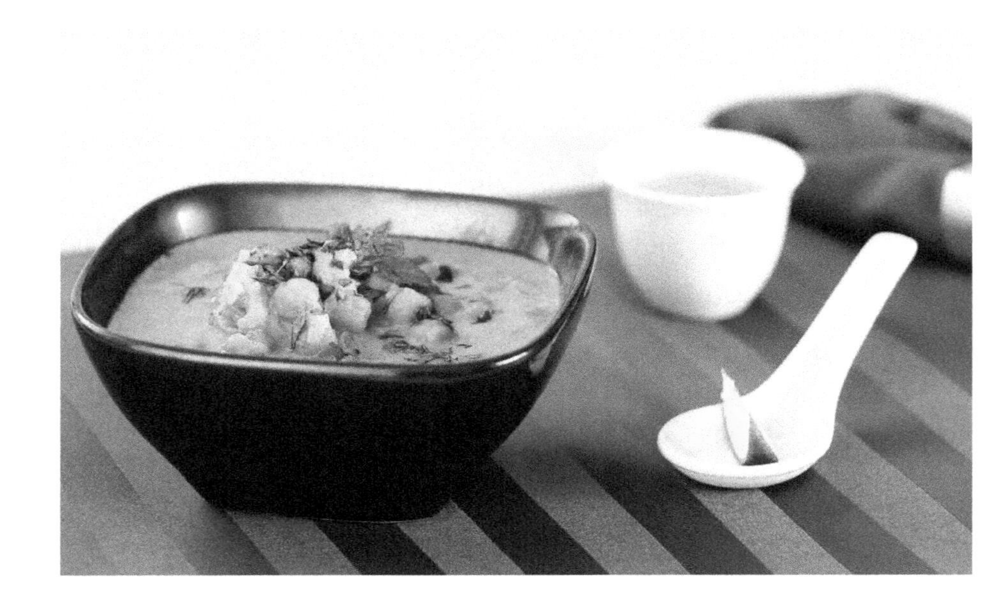

Chicken with Tomato and Lentils

Prep time: 10 minutes I **Cooking time:** 25 minutes I **Servings:** 4

Ingredients:

- 1 cup tomatoes, chopped
- Black pepper to the taste
- 1 tablespoon chipotle paste
- 1 pound chicken breast, skinless, boneless and cubed
- 2 cups lentils, cooked and drained
- ½ tablespoon olive oil
- 1 yellow onion, chopped
- 2 tablespoons cilantro, chopped

Directions:

1. Heat up a pan with the oil over medium heat, add the onion and chipotle paste, stir and sauté for 5 minutes.
2. Add the chicken, toss and brown for 5 minutes.
3. Add the rest of the ingredients, toss, cook everything for 15 minutes, divide into bowls and serve.

Nutrition facts per serving: calories 369, fat 17.6, fiber 9, carbs 44.8, protein 23.5

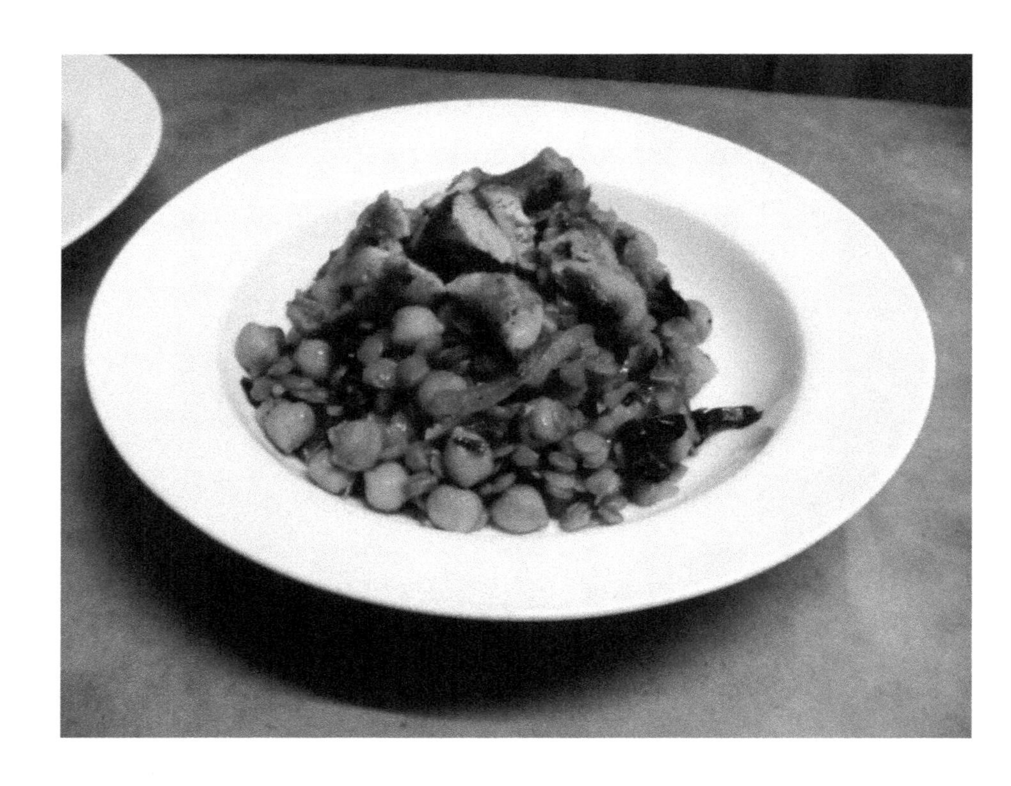

Balsamic Chicken and Cauliflower

Prep time: 5 minutes I **Cooking time:** 25 minutes I **Servings:** 4

Ingredients:

- 1 pound chicken breast, skinless, boneless and cubed
- 2 cups cauliflower florets
- 1 tablespoon olive oil
- 1 red onion, chopped
- 1 tablespoon balsamic vinegar
- ½ cup red bell pepper, chopped
- A pinch of black pepper
- 2 garlic cloves, minced
- ½ cup chicken stock
- 1 cup tomatoes, chopped

Directions:

1. Heat up a pan with the oil over medium-high heat, add the onion, garlic and the meat and brown for 5 minutes.
2. Add the rest of the ingredients, toss and cook over medium heat for 20 minutes.
3. Divide everything into bowls and serve for lunch.

Nutrition facts per serving: calories 366, fat 12, fiber 5.6, carbs 44.3, protein 23.7

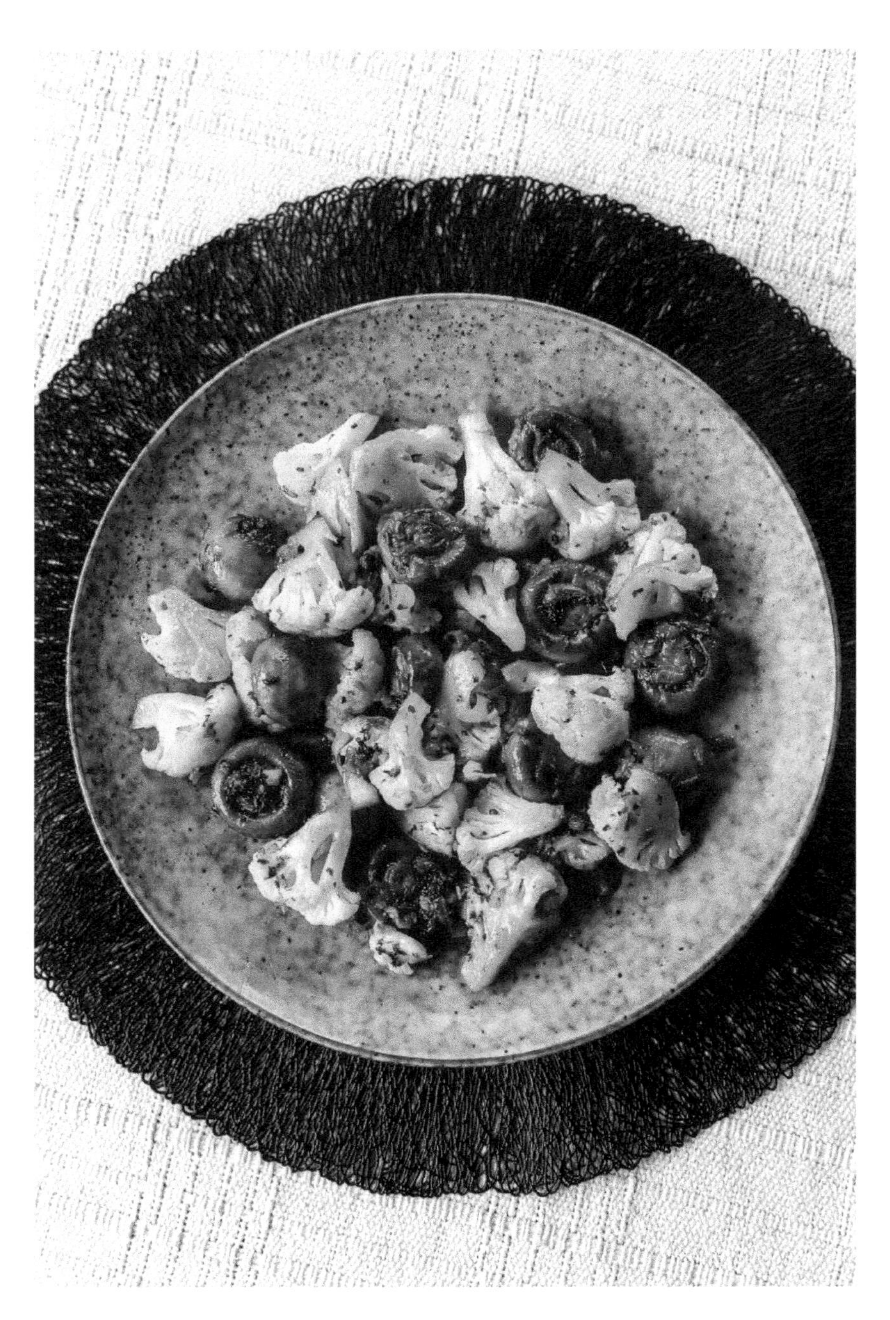

Basil Tomato Cream

Prep time: 10 minutes I **Cooking time:** 20 minutes I **Servings:** 4

Ingredients:

- 3 garlic cloves, minced
- 1 yellow onion, chopped
- 3 carrots, chopped
- 1 tablespoon olive oil
- 20 ounces roasted tomatoes, chopped
- 2 cup veggie stock
- 1 tablespoon basil, dried
- 1 cup coconut cream
- A pinch of black pepper

Directions:

1. Heat up a pot with the oil over medium heat, add the onion and the garlic and sauté for 5 minutes.
2. Add the rest of the ingredients, stir, bring to a simmer, cook for 15 minutes, blend the soup using an immersion blender, divide into bowls and serve for lunch.

Nutrition facts per serving: calories 244, fat 17.8, fiber 4.7, carbs 18.6, protein 3.8

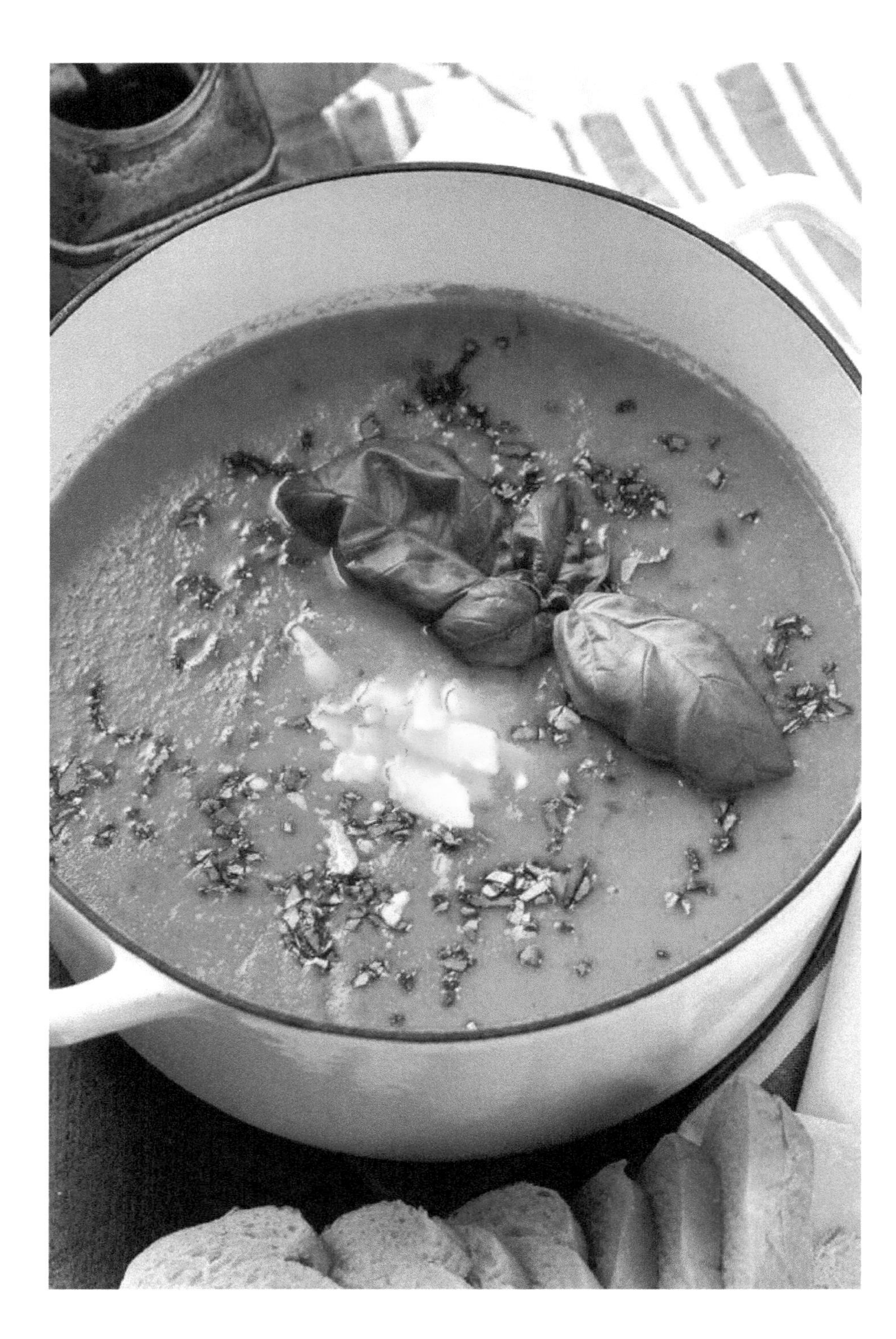

Herbed Pork Mix

Prep time: 10 minutes I **Cooking time:** 30 minutes I **Servings:** 4

Ingredients:

- 4 pork chops, boneless
- 1 pound sweet potatoes, peeled and cut into wedges
- 1 tablespoon olive oil
- 1 cup vegetable stock
- A pinch of black pepper
- 1 teaspoon oregano, dried
- 1 teaspoon rosemary, dried
- 1 teaspoon basil, dried

Directions:

1. Heat up a pan with the oil over medium-high heat, add the pork chops and cook them for 4 minutes on each side.
2. Add the sweet potatoes and the rest of the ingredients, put the lid on and cook over medium heat for 20 minutes more stirring from time to time.
3. Divide everything between plates and serve.

Nutrition facts per serving: calories 424, fat 23.7, fiber 5.1, carbs 32.3, protein 19.9

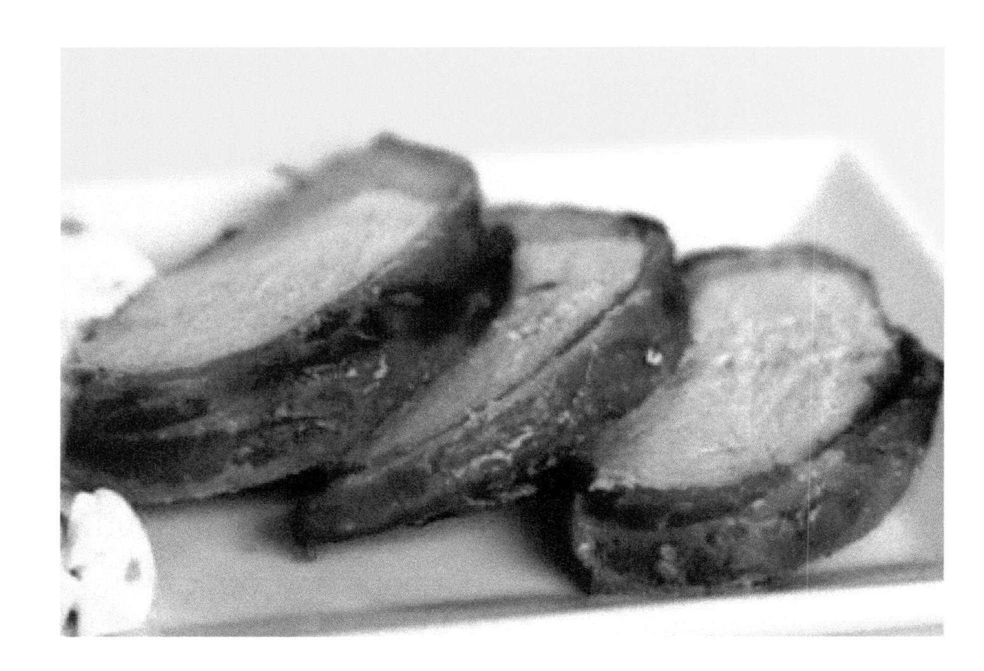

Trout Soup

Prep time: 10 minutes I **Cooking time:** 25 minutes I **Servings:** 4

Ingredients:

- 1 yellow onion, chopped
- 12 cups fish stock
- 1 pound carrots, sliced
- 1 pound trout fillets, boneless, skinless and cubed
- 1 tablespoon sweet paprika
- 1 cup tomatoes, cubed
- 1 tablespoon olive oil
- Black pepper to the taste

Directions:

1. Heat up a pot with the oil over medium-high heat, add the onion, stir and sauté for 5 minutes.
2. Add the fish, carrots and the rest of the ingredients, bring to a simmer and cook over medium heat for 20 minutes.
3. Ladle the soup into bowls and serve.

Nutrition facts per serving: calories 361, fat 13.4, fiber 4.6, carbs 164, protein 44.1

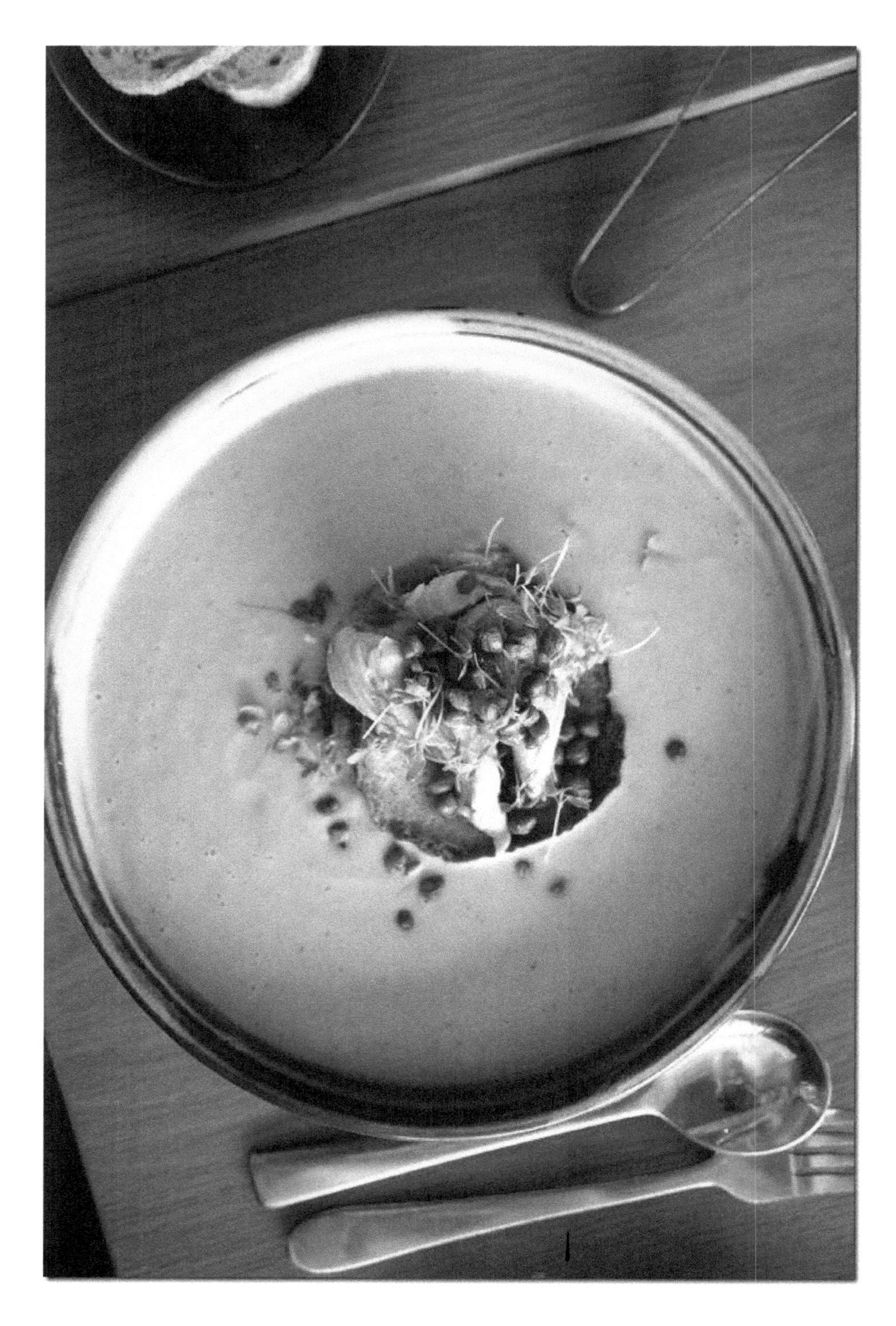

Turkey and Fennel Pan

Prep time: 10 minutes I **Cooking time:** 45 minutes I **Servings:** 4

Ingredients:

- 1 turkey breast, skinless, boneless and cubed
- 2 fennel bulbs, sliced
- 1 tablespoon olive oil
- 2 bay leaves
- 1 yellow onion, chopped
- 1 cup tomatoes, chopped
- 2 cup beef stock
- 3 garlic cloves, chopped
- Black pepper to the taste

Directions:

1. Heat up a pan with the oil over medium heat, add the onion and the meat and brown for 5 minutes.
2. Add the fennel and the rest of the ingredients, bring to a simmer and cook over medium heat for 40 minutes, stirring from time to time.
3. Divide the stew into bowls and serve.

Nutrition facts per serving: calories 371, fat 12.8, fiber 5.3, carbs 16.7, protein 11.9

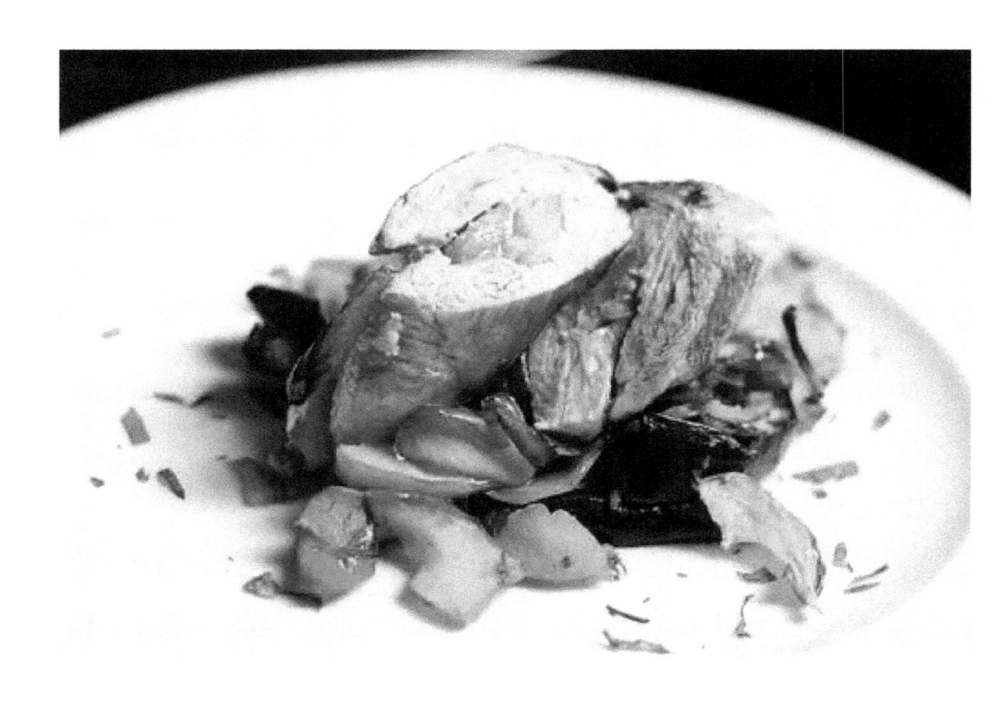

Cilantro Eggplant and Onion Soup

Prep time: 10 minutes I **Cooking time:** 30 minutes I **Servings:** 4

Ingredients:

- 2 big eggplants, roughly cubed
- 1 quart veggie stock
- 2 tablespoons tomato pasta
- 1 red onion, chopped
- 1 tablespoon olive oil
- 1 tablespoon cilantro, chopped
- A pinch of black pepper

Directions:

1. Heat up a pot with the oil over medium heat, add the onion, stir and sauté for 5 minutes.
2. Add the eggplants and the other ingredients, bring to a simmer over medium heat, cook for 25 minutes, divide into bowls and serve.

Nutrition facts per serving: calories 335, fat 14.4, fiber 5, carbs 16.1, protein 8.4

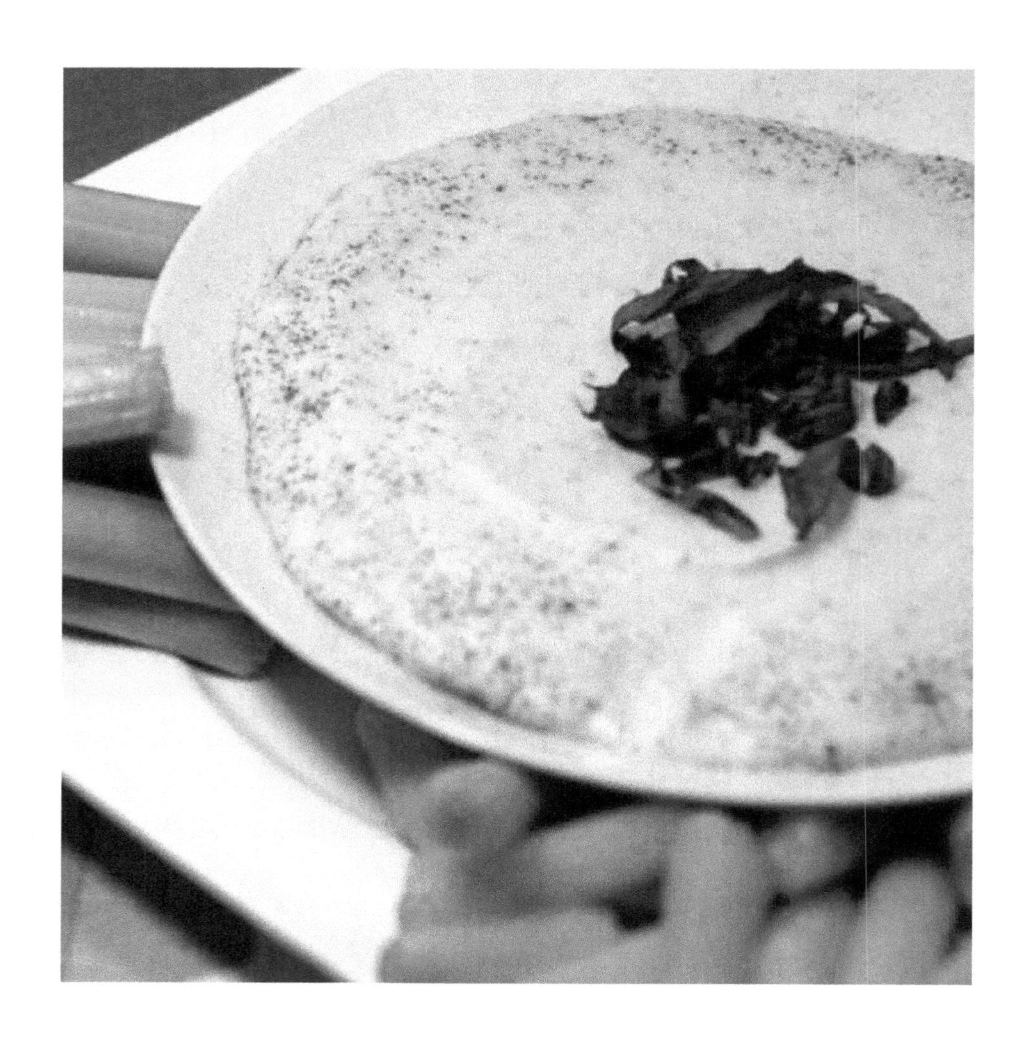

Coconut Onion and Potatoes Cream

Prep time: 10 minutes I **Cooking time:** 25 minutes I **Servings:** 4

Ingredients:

- 4 cups veggie stock
- 2 tablespoons avocado oil
- 2 sweet potatoes, peeled and cubed
- 2 yellow onions, chopped
- 2 garlic cloves, minced
- 1 cup coconut milk
- A pinch of black pepper
- ½ teaspoon basil, chopped

Directions:

1. Heat up a pot with the oil over medium heat, add the onion and the garlic, stir and sauté for 5 minutes.
2. Add the sweet potatoes and the rest of the ingredients, bring to a simmer and cook over medium heat for 20 minutes.
3. Blend the soup using an immersion blender, ladle into bowls and serve for lunch.

Nutrition facts per serving: calories 303, fat 14.4, fiber 4, carbs 9.8, protein 4.5

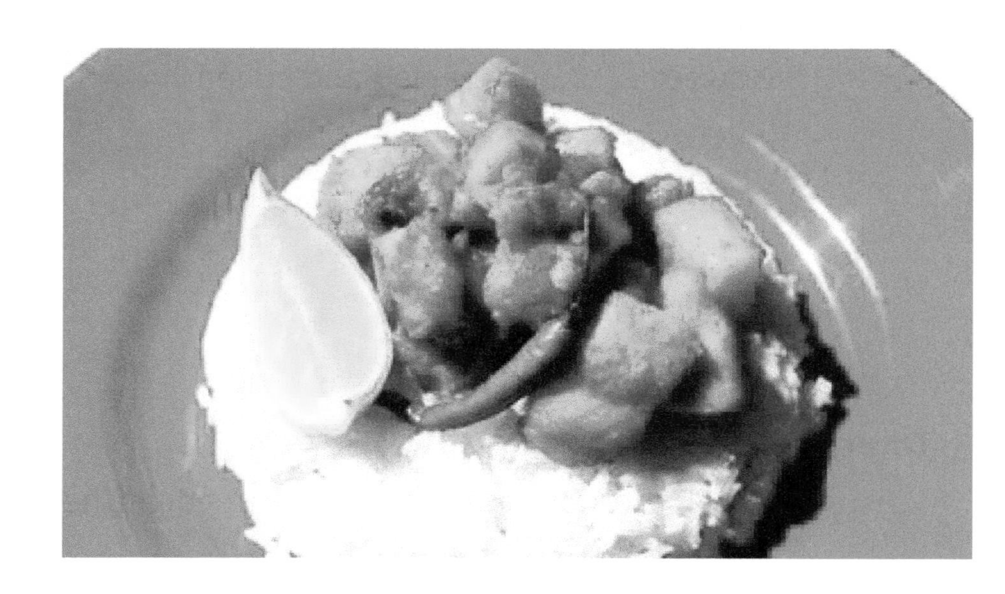

Hot Lime Chicken and Veggies Soup

Prep time: 10 minutes I **Cooking time:** 30 minutes I **Servings:** 4

Ingredients:

- 1 quart veggie stock
- 1 tablespoon ginger, grated
- 1 yellow onion, chopped
- 1 tablespoon olive oil
- 1 pound chicken breast, skinless, boneless and cubed
- ½ pound white mushrooms, sliced
- 4 red chilies, chopped
- ¼ cup lime juice
- ¼ cup cilantro, chopped
- A pinch of black pepper

Directions:

1. Heat up a pot with the oil over medium heat, add the onion, ginger, chilies and the meat, stir and brown for 5 minutes.
2. Add the mushrooms, stir and cook for 5 minutes more.
3. Add the rest of the ingredients, bring to a simmer and cook over medium heat for 20 minutes more.

4. Ladle the soup into bowls and serve right away.

Nutrition facts per serving: calories 226, fat 8.4, fiber 3.3, carbs 13.6, protein 28.2

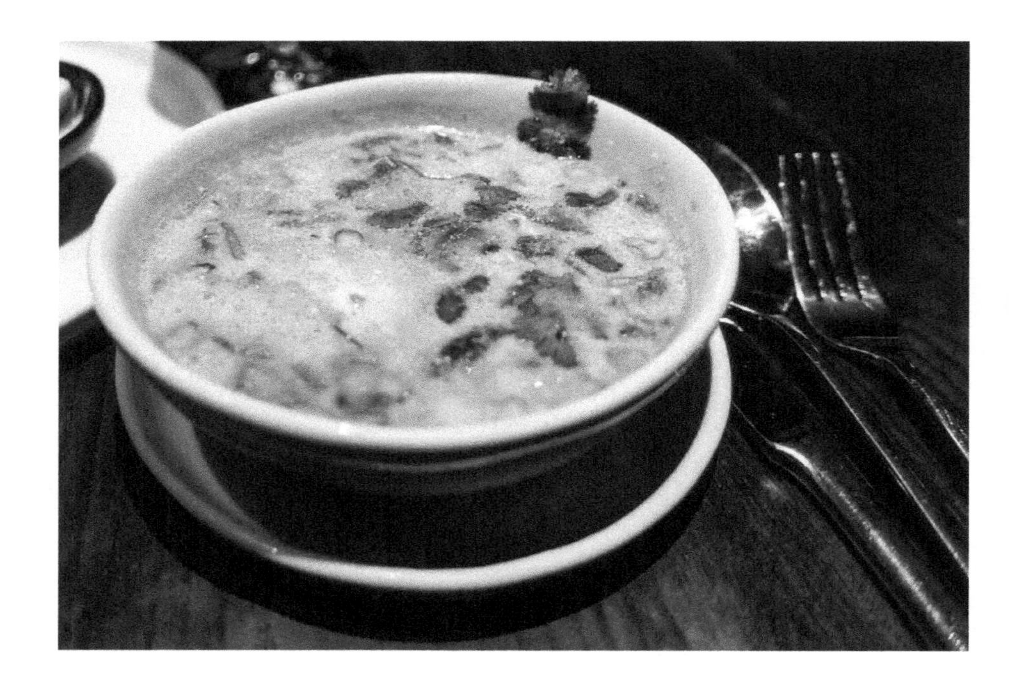

Thyme Salmon and Onion Mix

Prep time: 10 minutes I **Cooking time:** 20 minutes I **Servings:** 4

Ingredients:

- 4 salmon fillet, boneless
- 3 garlic cloves, minced
- 1 yellow onion, chopped
- Black pepper to the taste
- 2 tablespoons olive oil
- Juice of 1 lime
- 1 tablespoon lime zest, grated
- 1 tablespoon thyme, chopped

Directions:

5. Heat up a pan with the oil over medium-high heat, add the onion and garlic, stir and sauté for 5 minutes.
6. Add the fish and cook it for 3 minutes on each side.
7. Add the rest of the ingredients, cook everything for 10 minutes more, divide between plates and serve for lunch.

Nutrition facts per serving: calories 315, fat 18.1, fiber 1.1, carbs 4.9, protein 35.1

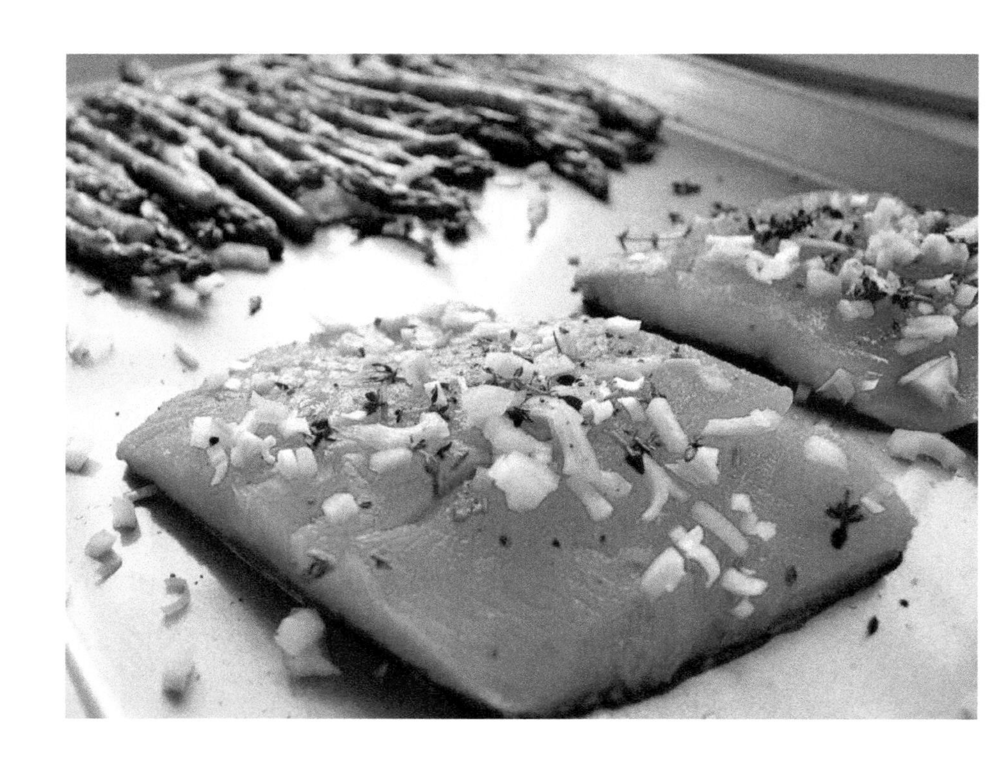

Potato, Tomato and Spinach Salad

Prep time: 10 minutes I **Cooking time:** 20 minutes I **Servings:** 4

Ingredients:

- 2 tomatoes, chopped
- 2 avocados, pitted and chopped
- 2 cups baby spinach
- 2 scallions, chopped
- 1 pound gold potatoes, boiled, peeled and cut into wedges
- 1 tablespoon olive oil
- 1 tablespoon lemon juice
- 1 yellow onion, chopped
- 2 garlic cloves, minced
- Black pepper to the taste
- 1 bunch cilantro, chopped

Directions:

1. Heat up a pan with the oil over medium-high heat, add the onion, scallions and the garlic, stir and sauté for 5 minutes.
2. Add the potatoes, toss gently and cook for 5 minutes more.

3. Add the rest of the ingredients, toss, cook over medium heat for 10 minutes more, divide into bowls and serve for lunch.

Nutrition facts per serving: calories 342, fat 23.4, fiber 11.7, carbs 33.5, protein 5

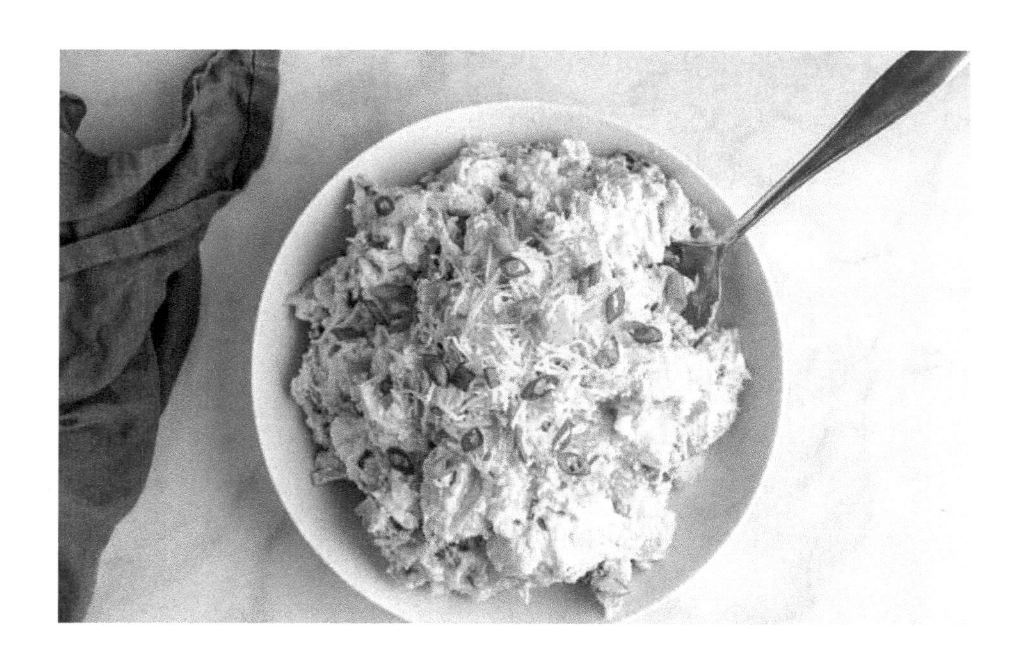

Ground Beef Pan

Prep time: 10 minutes I **Cooking time:** 20 minutes I **Servings:** 4

Ingredients:

- 1 pound beef, ground
- 1 red onion, chopped
- 1 tablespoon olive oil
- 1 cup cherry tomatoes, halved
- ½ red bell pepper, chopped
- Black pepper to the taste
- 1 tablespoon chives, chopped
- 1 tablespoon rosemary, chopped
- 3 tablespoons beef stock

Directions:

1. Heat up a pan with the oil over medium heat, add the onion and the bell pepper, stir and sauté for 5 minutes.
2. Add the meat, stir and brown it for another 5 minutes.
3. Add the rest of the ingredients, toss, cook for 10 minutes, divide into bowls and serve for lunch.

Nutrition facts per serving: calories 320, fat 11.3, fiber 4.4, carbs 18.4, protein 9

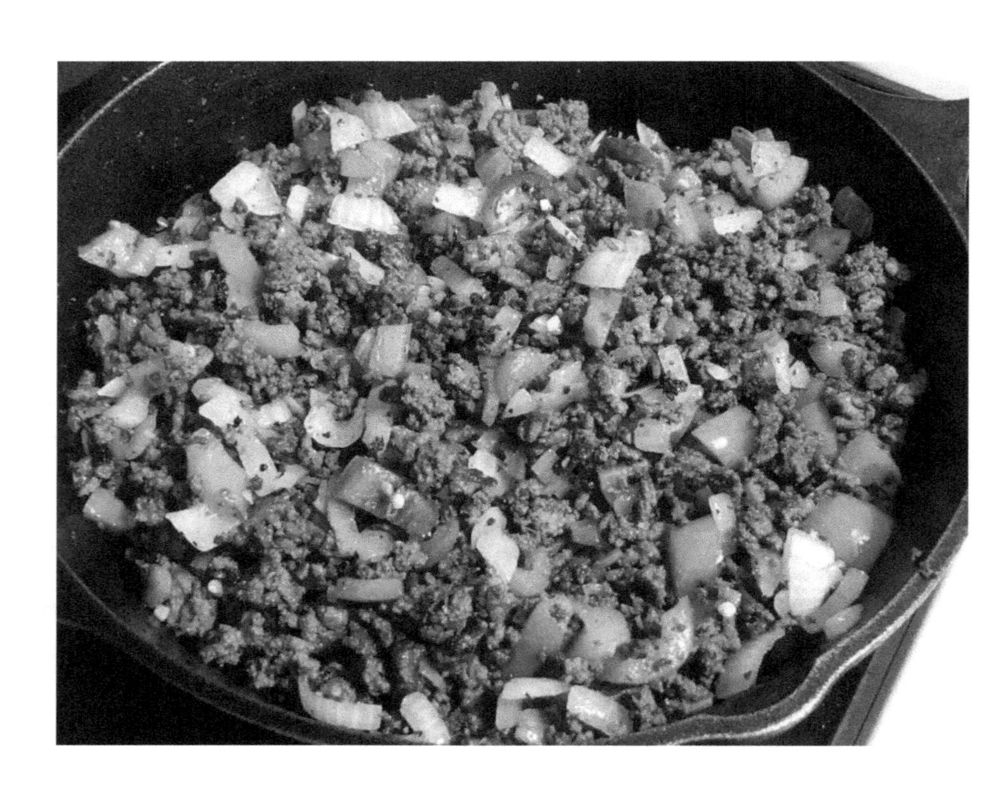

Lightning Source UK Ltd.
Milton Keynes UK
UKHW050828291222
414375UK00005B/29